Praise for

## *Could It Be . . . Perimenopause?*

"Perimenopause is one of the most important issues facing women of my age group. . . . Many gynecologists are more comfortable dealing with surgical issues, contraception, and pregnancy than with the very difficult, nebulous subject of perimenopause. Dr. Goldstein is one of the few who address a very real health problem that afflicts almost every woman."

— Beryl Benacerraf, M.D., Clinical Professor of Obstetrics, Gynecology and Reproductive Biology and Radiology, Harvard Medical School

"Could it be . . . *I feel better* after reading Dr. Goldstein's book! Clear, understandable information on a subject we baby boomers need to know about now."

— Carol Levin, Founder and Director, Optimum Wellness Now Women's Health Support Group, New York University

"This clearly written and immensely readable book makes accessible to all women a wealth of information about this phase of feminine development. Dr. Goldstein and Ms. Ashner describe perimenopause in terms of the physiological changes that occur, and they explore with great sensitivity the effects that these changes have on our emotions, thought processes, and sexuality. This information, combined with the practical, useful coping strategies they suggest, can be an enormously powerful tool for women to use in transforming their experience of perimenopause."

— Dr. Carla Solomon, Clinical Psychologist and Psychoanalyst; Member, The New York Psychoanalytic Institute and Society

"Every woman between the ages of thirty-five and fifty should read this book. Dr. Goldstein has given women valuable information and options for our peace of mind and well-being."

— Elisabeth Halfpapp, Fitness Director and Vice-President, Lotte Berk Method Limited

Also by Steven R. Goldstein, M.D., and Laurie Ashner

*The Estrogen Alternative: What Every Woman Needs to Know About Hormone Replacement Therapy and SERMs, the New Estrogen Substitutes*

Also by Laurie Ashner

*When Parents Love Too Much*
*Resonance: The New Chemistry of Love*
*When Is Enough, Enough? What You Can Do if You Never Feel Satisfied*

# Could It Be . . . Perimenopause?

---

HOW WOMEN 35–50 CAN OVERCOME FORGETFULNESS,
MOOD SWINGS, INSOMNIA, WEIGHT GAIN,
SEXUAL DYSFUNCTION, AND OTHER TELLTALE SIGNS
OF HORMONAL IMBALANCE

---

*Steven R. Goldstein, M.D.,*
*and Laurie Ashner*

Little, Brown and Company
BOSTON   NEW YORK   LONDON

Originally published in hardcover by Little, Brown and Company, 1998
First paperback edition, 2000

The information in this book is not intended and should not be construed as medical advice. If you need medical attention, please seek the advice of your own health practitioner. You should have your health professional check your condition before making any changes in an existing treatment program.

Library of Congress Cataloging-in-Publication Data

Goldstein, Steven R.
    Could it be . . . perimenopause? : how women 35–50 can overcome forgetfulness, mood swings, insomnia, weight gain, sexual dysfunction, and other telltale signs of hormonal imbalance / Steven R. Goldstein and Laurie Ashner. — 1st ed.
        p.   cm.
    Includes index.
    ISBN 0-316-31898-1 (hc) / 0-316-31945-7 (pb)
    1. Perimenopause — Popular works.   I. Ashner, Laurie.   II. Title.
    RG188.G64   1998
    618.1'75 — dc21                                                                98-3104

10 9 8 7 6 5 4 3

Q-FF

Printed in the United States of America

# CONTENTS

FOREWORD                                                                          *ix*

ACKNOWLEDGMENTS                                                                    *xi*

INTRODUCTION                                                                        *3*

1   *It's Not All in Your Head: What Those Subtle Symptoms Mean and*
    *What You Can Do About Them*                                                   *10*

2   *A Closer Look at Your Symptoms*                                               *23*

3   *You Don't Have to Feel This Way*                                             *46*

4   *Should You Treat Your Symptoms Naturally?*                                    *68*

5   *Will You Gain Ten Pounds During Perimenopause?: The Secret to*
    *Weight Control During Transition*                                            *87*

6   *Rx for Black Moods and Other Symptoms*                                       *103*

7   *How to Stay Out of the O.R.*                                                 *118*

8   *How to Get the Most from Medical Science — While Avoiding the Worst*         *136*

9   *Sex, Sexuality, and Fertility*                                              *152*

10  *Menopause: How Will You Know It When You Get There?*                        *172*

11  *Plain Talk About Estrogen*                                                  *188*

12  *Getting Support Twenty-four Hours a Day*                                    *201*

13  *Your Emotions: Mind-sets That Matter*                                       *210*

EPILOGUE: MEDICINE IN THE NEW MILLENNIUM                                          222

APPENDIX                                                                          229

INDEX                                                                             235

# FOREWORD

At one time *menopause* was a hated word — it described the person as "beginning to be old." Now, instead it describes the beginning of the second half of an experienced and settled woman's life. *Perimenopause* is still a frightening word to many women, some of whom are just ending their thirties and often just contemplating their life's goals.

This book explains that perimenopause is only a poorly chosen word for a transitional hormonal stage that may be temporary and may occur many years before true menopause. In fact, a recent scientific study showed that the range of normal for the duration of perimenopause varies from four to fifteen years!

Until now, this era in the female life cycle has not been well understood and in fact has been ignored both in the literature and in clinical practice despite the severe impact on a patient's quality of life. Today's perimenopausal woman has neither the time nor the patience to go through four to fifteen years of symptoms without relief.

Unlike menopause, which can be strictly defined and proven with laboratory tests, perimenopause has far more fluctuation and is actually defined as "irregularly irregular" hormone levels. The perimenopausal process is highly individualized, with great variation from woman to woman. At last, Dr. Goldstein has explained this unrecognized, understudied, and undertreated condition. He clarifies the details and specific complaints and symptoms that can help each woman decide if her problem is perimenopause. He has also done a great job of bringing the subject of birth-control pills into the twenty-first century. Women who haven't kept up with the science of oral contraceptives need to know how much has changed. Dr. Goldstein points out the lower doses, flexible schedules, and some surprising advantages (e.g., great decreases in incidence of ovarian and endometrial cancer) that these medications now have. He has also updated a host of other topics, including the most accurate, complete, and scientific information on "natural" products. He also discusses the best way to surf the Internet for information on perimenopause, the latest information on "designer estrogens," and in general smooths this difficult transition. This is an accurate, up-to-date, thoroughly readable and sympathetic guide, one I would heartily recommend to any woman undergoing "the change before the change."

Lila E. Nachtigall, M.D.

# ACKNOWLEDGMENTS

A little more than a decade ago I wrote the acknowledgments to the first of three medical texts I have authored. I said then that I savored to the very last the task of thanking all those who helped me get to where I was. I feel the same way today. Rarely does one get an opportunity to publicly and in writing tell people who matter "Thank you." Thus, I would like to thank Laurie Ashner, for being bright and vivacious, an outstanding writer, and, thank God, a quick read, and above all for her never-ending sense of humor; Jean Naggar, my agent, for her enthusiasm, expertise, and for introducing me to Laurie; Mike Frankfurt of Frankfurt Garbus, not only because he taught me how to run marathons and because he is my friend, but also for looking over my legal contracts; Robert F. Porges, M.D., and Charles Lockwood, M.D., my previous and current academic chairmen and friends, who maintain an environment at NYU Medical Center where someone like me can produce the things I have and, I hope, will continue to produce; Ken Kaplan, M.D., and the doctors who assist him, Gary Mucciolo, M.D., Andy Gardner, M.D., Meredith Halpern, M.D., Yvette Martes, M.D., Scott Smilen, M.D., and Michael Silverstein, M.D., without whose able-bodied coverage of my practice this work and all my academic life could not function; Camille Horan, RDMS, Jon Snyder, M.D., and Lisa Schwartz, M.D., my Gyn Ultrasound colleagues, to whom I owe so much; Lila Nachtigall, M.D., my friend, colleague, teacher, and partner, who has taught me so much; my staff: Karen Bollaert, Christine Sweeney, Concetta Tepe, Ellen Bloom, and Juanita Castro, who are so wonderful to my patients, and who put up with me and keep me pointed in the right direction; my patients, who really deserve much of the credit for teaching me so much of what I have come to know and understand; my parents, Joseph and Margery Goldstein, who live on in my heart; my brother, Howard S. Goldstein, M.D., for being the best big brother and sounding board I could ever hope for; my children, Phoebe and Luke, for making a place in eternity for me and enriching my life in uncountable ways; and most of all my wife, Kathy Dillon Goldstein, the person I have dedicated this book to, for changing my life in so many positive ways that continue to unfold every day.

Steven R. Goldstein, M.D.

I would like to thank Karen Boos and Nancy Block, two women who know how to get the job done right, for their help in getting these concepts into a manuscript; Susan Piser, for her insights into the psychological ramifications of perimenopause; Alice Stamm, for teaching me how useful the Internet can be for women in perimenopause; Mark and Martha Rubenstein, for the insight and the web site; the patients of Dr. Goldstein who were willing to speak candidly to me for hours and whose experiences are so much a part of this book; my in-laws, Ed and Marion Meyerson, who have always encouraged my writing; Ellen Gradman, Noni George, J. K., Mary Wells, Carrie Worley, Marcie and Howard Tilkin, and Ellie Sigel, for their friendship and love — without you it wouldn't have happened. A special thanks to my agent, Jean Naggar, for introducing me to Dr. Steven Goldstein and the exciting year that followed.

Laurie Ashner

# Could It Be . . . Perimenopause?

# INTRODUCTION

When it began, Susan,* forty-two, barely noticed. She was at an art fair when she ran into a man who had recently joined her division at work. She started to introduce him to her husband. "Suddenly the guy's name was a complete blank," she says. "But I figured so what? It was embarrassing, but I hardly knew him."

When she started to forget phone numbers, she worried. "I always remembered phone numbers. I was proud of that. Now I'd dial and the number would be on the tip of my tongue — and stay there."

She thought it was nerves. "I felt run-down, irritated, overall lousy. Between work and getting my daughter ready to go to school for the first time in the fall, there was a lot on my mind. No wonder I was walking into rooms and forgetting why I entered them."

Then one Saturday morning, standing in line to get cash for her groceries, she forgot her ATM number. "I thought, 'How can you forget four numbers you've used twice a week for five years?' What was happening to me?

"What haunted me was that I have a family history of Alzheimer's, although not my parents or grandparents. But the idea that I might be showing some early signs terrified me.

"I went to the library. I hid the books on Alzheimer's in the back of the pantry where my husband and daughter would never stumble on them."

---

* The stories in this book are based on the experiences of actual people, but the names and circumstances have been altered to ensure confidentiality.

When Susan came to my office, it was for an annual gynecological exam. She looked tired and admitted that she wasn't sleeping well. She hadn't confided her fears to anyone. She told me that since her fortieth birthday her menses had become less regular and now ranged from twenty-two to forty days apart. Susan had no idea that the changes in her menstrual cycle could be related to her bouts of forgetfulness. Nor did she know how quickly proper treatment would restore her memory.

Today Susan takes Loestrin, an ultra-low-dose birth-control pill specifically designed for women over forty. Although her breasts are a little more tender, her memory has improved, and she is greatly relieved.

Amy, forty-four, began to realize that there were only about eight to ten days of every month when she felt good. On those days she was hopeful. Grounded. Optimistic. Peaceful.

The other days? A roller coaster of swollen, sore breasts, jeans that wouldn't zip, hunger that nothing assuaged. Add that to a dark, evil-feeling depression that mysteriously lifted its dead weight the day after she got her period.

"I've had PMS in the past," she told me, "gotten a little cranky, but never anything like this. I can't concentrate. My thoughts are always racing. My allergist told me that the pollen count has been high; it makes people feel spacy. He said I should exercise indoors."

But then something strange happened one night. "I was having dinner with a friend at a new restaurant. One minute we were talking and everything was fine. Then I started to feel strange, like I was eight feet above everyone in the room. My pulse quickened; my heart pounded. I thought, '*I've got to get out of here. Now.*' We left the restaurant before the food came.

"My sister told me about hypoglycemia. I had a test. Nothing. My internist shook his head and asked me if there was anything going on at home. I told him that Jack and I had been together for over six years, that we weren't married but we were happy. He gave me a look like he didn't quite believe me. Why weren't we married? he wanted to know. As if that had anything to do with it! He recommended Prozac. He felt I was depressed."

It wasn't the pollen count. It wasn't her subconscious mind telling her she should get married. And she didn't need Prozac.

After a thorough examination, I diagnosed Amy as "ogligo ovulatory," which means that she was only ovulating sporadically. Instead of Prozac, she went on Provera, a form of progesterone that functions like the hormone the body would produce normally when a woman ovulates.

After two months she has never felt better. Her energy is high, concentration is back to where it was, and the attacks of anxiety have diminished.

When Lynne, forty-seven, went for her annual exam, she tried to discuss the many differences she was experiencing in her health recently — subtle and hard to pinpoint, but very definite differences that when added up were making her feel unlike her natural self.

She'd gotten her last period weeks before she expected it, and it caught her at work, completely unprepared. "It reminded me of junior high, having to search the halls for an understanding teacher or someone who could loan me a tampon or a pad."

Her doctor listened carefully. "He said that since I was still having periods, there was no reason to do hormone levels. Then he told me that since my daughter was a teenager and I probably would not be planning any more children, I might as well have a hysterectomy. His suggestion was 'See if it helps.' I stood there, stunned."

There was every reason to "do hormone levels" (which I did) and no reason for a hysterectomy. I gave Lynne a detailed explanation of what was happening inside her body and options she could take if her symptoms did not improve. It was enough to dispel her worries.

It is not uncommon to hear stories like this. If you are a woman in your late thirties or forties and you are experiencing symptoms like those Amy, Lynne, and Susan experienced — sleep disturbances, free-floating anxiety, inability to concentrate, forgetfulness, mood swings — you need to know that this is very likely not all in your head.

There probably *is* something physical happening here. It isn't that your youngest is entering high school, or there's been an upheaval at the office, or your husband is having an affair, or you've broken off a relationship. These symptoms may be related to destabilizing estrogen levels and a decrease in ovulation.

You are entering a stage known as perimenopause, which begins about a decade before the onset of actual menopause. And you are far from alone. In the year 2000, 21.2 million women in this country will enter perimenopause. The onset of actual menopause will be far from their minds, and will, in most cases, be many years away physically. Yet, even though every woman will go through perimenopause, it is one of the least understood, most misdiagnosed, and most confounding stages in a woman's life.

I told this to a patient recently who said, "Dr. Goldstein, I'm thirty-nine years old. I don't want to even hear the word *menopause*, let alone think about it. I'm trying to have another baby. I'm still young. Don't talk to me about menopause."

It is essential to understand that we are not talking about "early menopause," which is why current books available on menopause don't help and often confuse, depress, or frighten younger women. Early menopause means that you stop menstruating completely for a period of at least twelve months, and that this occurs before the age of forty-five.

What you're experiencing is not menopause and not PMS (premenstrual syndrome). This book is about a distinct stage with symptoms and realities of its own that responds to specialized health-care strategies.

Years ago I came to realize that it is the decade *before* menopause that needs my patients' full attention. By the time you are menopausal, it's too late. For many, many women, the decade before menopause can be a stormy, disruptive transition from regular cyclic menses and the predictable symptoms that go along with it to what we know of as menopause.

Gail Sheehy, in her book *The Silent Passage,* wrote that most women still don't realize that the peak of emotional symptoms and bleeding problems occurs years before the actual event of menopause. Sheehy called menopause "the calm after the storm." This book is about the storm. It will educate you about what you are experiencing, and that knowledge will become personal power. You will have the facts you need to make clear choices about medicinal therapies that are available to you. You will know what is going on with your body both physically and psychologically. You will learn about healthy lifestyle choices — exercise, diet, nutrition, vitamins, the power of a positive outlook — that you can begin to make today that will have far-reaching ramifications for your overall health. You will learn what my patients have learned: *Just knowing what's going on inside your body may be enough to make a real difference in the way you feel.*

Chances are if you are reading this book, you already know that something new is happening to you. But it probably isn't menopause. There is a clear medical distinction between the symptoms of a lack of estrogen — the hallmark of menopause — and the more subtle symptoms of the transitional phase, which can hit some women as young as their late thirties. To give women in transition estrogen supplements and treat them as if they are in the midst of early menopause is an all-too-frequent misdiagnosis, with discomfiting, and sometimes harmful, results.

While much has been written about the effects a woman experiences when she no longer produces estrogen, it is *fluctuating* levels of estrogen without progesterone that cause the symptoms in the decade prior to menopause. But these symptoms needn't be scary or mysterious or something women are stuck with. There are many things any woman can do to make the years of transition much less disruptive.

The chapters that follow answer the questions my patients have asked most frequently about perimenopause, including:

- How can a menstrual cycle that swings from twenty-four days to thirty-six days to twenty-two days be the real culprit behind a sequence of up times and times when you feel moody, tense, and unable to concentrate?

- What specific medical treatments can give you the upper hand — and the most benefits?
- What's the truth about weight gain during this stage? As one woman put it, "Is the remainder of my life going to be a fork, a lettuce leaf, and Premarin on the side?"
- How can you maintain your equilibrium and make this transition in your body less disruptive?
- What exactly is going on in your body? What hormones are you making and in what quantity, and what are you becoming deficient in? Why do these hormones matter?
- What do you do about missing periods, gushing periods, and periods that never seem to end?
- What are the strongest natural remedies for mood swings, anxiety, fatigue, and other symptoms that make you feel out of balance?
- How can you stay out of the operating room and the emergency room?
- What's the bottom line on estrogen? Should you replace this hormone with drugs once your body no longer produces it naturally?
- What does medical science have to offer for the changes in sex drive you may be experiencing?
- What is the truth about dong quai, yam roots, soy, black cohosh, and other "natural" remedies that thousands of women are buying at health-food stores?
- What are the myths and realities about cancer in the new millennium?
- What's the real essence of the arguments for and against going back on the Pill in your forties?
- What can you do to boost your vitality and improve your mental health?

Using case examples, I will explain to you why certain people are more vulnerable to disequilibrium than others. I will explore the misguided health strategies that harm you more than they help you. I will answer the questions women are sometimes afraid to ask their doctors.

If you see yourself clearly and unmistakably in the pages that follow, you'll have a no-nonsense guide to exchanging chronic subtle symptoms for greater vitality and health.

# 1

# IT'S NOT ALL IN YOUR HEAD
## What Those Subtle Symptoms Mean and What You Can Do About Them

When it first starts to happen to you, the symptoms are so subtle that by the time you start to worry, they're often gone. You mention your anxiety, your fatigue, your bouts of forgetfulness to your friends. They nod knowingly. They've had them too. Your husband says *he's* had them. He doesn't worry; why should you?

But still, there are these differences in the way you feel, these annoying symptoms. You think about making an appointment to see your doctor. But what will you say? That you feel vaguely anxious? That you're suddenly having trouble putting names with faces? That you've taken to going to bed an hour before your husband when you aren't even tired to avoid another argument over sex?

You wonder, "Maybe this is all in my head."

*I told my sister that I'd be on the way to school to pick my daughter up and I'd forget where I was going and why. She just said, "Oh, that happens to me too. You're just stressed out."*

*I gained eight pounds in a matter of months. I would go out and run for an hour, and the next day the scale would tell me I'd gained five pounds. No one believed me when I said I watched everything I ate and exercised three times a week. I started to wonder if this was the way it was going to be from now on: I'd spend my life eating salad and be enormous by the time I was forty-five.*

*My period would come all of a sudden, when I least expected it. It would last for two weeks. Then it wouldn't come for two months, and I'd freak, thinking I was pregnant. "Don't worry," my best friend told me, "I've never been regular."*

*I had absolutely no interest in sex. If I went the rest of my life and never had it again, that would be fine with me. My mood swings sent me to a marriage counselor. She kept asking me if I was angry with my husband. It didn't fit, and I told her so. She said it was clear I was out of touch with my feelings.*

The last thing you may attribute such symptoms to is subtle changes in your menstrual cycle, but they *are* related. In this chapter you will read about changes in the pattern of ovulation that most women experience in their late thirties and throughout their forties, and the effects of these changes on your emotional and physical well-being. When you fully understand these changes, you can do much to take charge of your body and regain a sense of equilibrium.

## Lighter, Heavier, Shorter, Longer — What Do Changes in Your Menstrual Cycle Mean?

This is what they taught you about your menstrual cycle in junior high school when you sat in the back of the classroom and giggled with the other girls: You make estrogen for two weeks, then you ovulate, then you make progesterone for two weeks. One of God's givens is that two weeks after ovulation, you will get a menses. So the only thing that's variable is how long before you ovulate.

What they didn't explain is that over a lifetime, there are three places you can be:

You can be living in this seventh-grade-health-class menstrual cycle. Or you can be in menopause, when you don't make any estrogen or progesterone — menstruation stops. Or you can be in the third place. There will be a time, variable in length, beginning as early as your late thirties or any time throughout your forties, when you will find yourself between these two places. Think of it as transition.

## Irregular Is What's Regular During Transition

Irregular is regular at this time of your life. Shorter, longer, lighter, heavier, the character of your period can change so much during perimenopause that you wonder, Is this normal?

I have patients who are at my office immediately when their cycle is off. But the majority of women I see may have great irregularity to their bleeding cycle, although they may not be aware of it. The change is often subtle. Especially if you aren't worried about getting pregnant, you don't always notice if your period is a few days late or a few days early.

Marilyn, forty-five, for example, came in for an annual exam. Her complaint? "I'm having horrible PMS. I've never, ever had a problem before, not even cramps in high school. Now I have about one week a month where I'm symptom free, where my breasts don't ache, where I don't want to slaughter the newspaper guy because he's out of the *New York Times.*"

I asked her if she'd noticed any changes in her menstrual cycle. She told me, "I've been a little irregular. But I'm not in a relationship right now, so I don't really think about if my period's late or early. I know I'm not pregnant."

She had jotted the dates down, however. We were able to map out her last six or seven periods. They had been 22 days, 27 days, 37 days, 38 days, 19 days, 27 days, and 21 days apart. The point was, though, that she had probably ovulated only twice in that interval.

One may think, "So what? If she isn't trying to get pregnant, what does it matter if she doesn't ovulate every month?"

Episodes of anovulation — cycles when you do not ovulate — are characterized by variable amounts of estrogen production without progesterone to balance it. This "imbalance" isn't dangerous (although unopposed estrogen for very long periods of time, which is unusual, may predispose women to hyperplasia [precancer] and sometimes cancer), but it is the basis of a host of symptoms that appear to be totally unrelated to your menstrual cycle.

## Estrogen, Progesterone, and Your Menstrual Cycle

Let's take a closer look at the hormones, estrogen and progesterone. Estrogen is made from follicles that develop each month in the ovaries. A follicle is a saclike structure inside the ovary that contains an egg. At the end of a cycle, if pregnancy does not ensue, the menstrual lining of the uterus is shed. The first day of the period begins day one of a new cycle. At that point, both ovaries recruit about a half dozen follicles under the influence of follicle stimulating hormone (FSH) from the pituitary gland in the brain. Around day nine, one follicle takes off geometrically and becomes the dominant follicle. It is a small (2¹/₂ cm) cystic structure prior to its bursting (i.e., ovulation). At midcycle (day fourteen), a surge of LH (luteinizing hormone) from the pituitary causes the follicle to rupture, releasing the ovum to be picked up by a fallopian tube.

The follicle is now known as the corpus luteum (Latin for "yellow body," because it looks yellow), and it begins to produce large amounts of progesterone. Progesterone causes the glands of the endometrium (the lining of the uterus) to become lush in preparation for receiving the fertilized egg. If no pregnancy ensues, estrogen and progesterone levels decrease and you get your period fourteen days after ovulation. Recall that the beginning of bleeding is day one of the new cycle.

Thus, in an idealized twenty-eight-day cycle you ovulate on day fourteen, and fourteen days later you get a menses. As you get older your cycle length will shorten to less than the classic twenty-eight days — often to twenty-four or twenty-five days — because women at this age begin to ovulate as early as day ten or day eleven. (If you ovulate on day ten you get a menses fourteen days later. Therefore, your cycle is ten plus fourteen, or twenty-four days.) The character of the actual menstrual bleed may remain the same, but the interval between bleeds shortens because of this earlier ovulation. Medical science does not have an explanation as to why older women begin to ovulate earlier, but it is a well-documented fact. However, some women will have a shortened postovulatory phase where ovulation still takes place at the proper time, but the period comes ten, eleven, or twelve days later instead of the classic fourteen days. This may be one of several reasons why fertility is diminishing in women of this age.

If your period has begun to come earlier than usual, it is generally because you've ovulated earlier. But this is not always the case. Marilyn, my patient, assumed that she was ovulating because she had her period. To most women, any bleeding from their vagina is their "period." But not all bleeding has been preceded by ovulation. During perimenopause, the egg-producing follicles in a woman's ovaries begin to become depleted, and those that remain become resistant to FSH (follicle stimulating hormone). Recall that FSH is the hormone that tells the ovary to start functioning. If nothing happens, the pituitary begins to pump out even more FSH. Without progesterone to trigger menstruation, the endometrium lining can keep building up.

When a woman has variable levels of estrogen, the lining of the uterus can be destabilized and will thus be shed. The woman feels she has had a period.

In the next chapter I will outline all the different scenarios of irregular bleeding that women can endure during perimenopause. For now, let's concentrate on irregularities that occur when you don't ovulate, the most frequent pattern.

## Unopposed Estrogen and Your Subtle Symptoms

When a woman does not ovulate, she makes no progesterone. If she does not ovulate and the estrogen level stays relatively constant, she will not bleed at all. When a woman goes eight, ten, twelve weeks without a period and is not pregnant, this is typical of anovulation with fairly constant estrogen levels.

How important is this lack of progesterone to balance out the estrogen? Researchers have found that when estrogen levels alone are rising, a host of physical symptoms can develop, including:

- Salt and fluid retention
- Low blood-sugar levels
- Blood clotting
- Fibroid tumor enhancement

- Altered thyroid hormone function (leading to weight gain and/or feelings of exhaustion)
- Increased production of body fat
- A sluggish, low-energy feeling

In addition, many women experience subtle psychological symptomatology that in the past has been chalked up to everything except fluctuating levels of unopposed estrogen. These symptoms include:

- Depression
- Free-floating anxiety
- Sleep disturbances
- Forgetfulness
- Changes in libido (i.e., less desire for sex than usual)
- Mood swings
- Inability to concentrate

A word of caution about these symptoms: There are a myriad of medical conditions that can cause you to feel tired and/or forgetful, anxious, etc. It's when doctors see a "family" of symptoms that occur following a specific pattern of events that we make a preliminary diagnosis. Not all of these symptoms are hormonally mediated. I have some of these symptoms, and I don't make any estrogen. But a significant number of women in their thirties, forties, and early fifties have symptoms that are related to levels of unopposed estrogen. What you undergo when this happens feels to many women like the reverse of adolescence.

Perimenopause is one of today's most misdiagnosed conditions. There are women who spend years making the rounds of internists, psychiatrists, neurologists, and other specialists, looking for an answer to the vague, often difficult-to-define changes in their bodies.

Karen, forty-two, tells a story that is a case in point: " 'I know exactly what you have,' this one psychiatrist told me. She spoke with such assurance that I started to feel hopeful. Here was someone who finally *knew*. 'They call it panic disorder,' she continued, and she read me a long list of symptoms of panic attacks.

"It fit, but somehow it didn't. True, I was waking up in the middle of the night. But the only panic I felt was fear over whether I'd be able to go back to sleep. Stressed out? Definitely. Learning that my ex-husband was getting remarried was a shock. I tried to connect that to the type of anxiety I was feeling several times a day, and it just didn't add up. I was actually happy for him.

"Then there was the day my new dining-room table was being delivered. The deliverymen scraped the entranceway, leaving a thick stripe of bare, brown drywall. I had a meltdown: tears, yelling, the whole thing. Two days later, my period came. I figured, okay, that's the deal, PMS. Still, my period was at least a week early, maybe more.

"I said as much to the psychiatrist. 'Well, stress can do that,' she told me. 'Some women skip periods for months when they are under this kind of stress.'

"I walked away with a prescription for Prozac in my purse, along with a bill for two hundred dollars and an appointment come back twice a week.

"The entire way home I thought, 'Prozac. Come on. I'm not that depressed.' When I told my sister I was going to throw the prescription out, she said, 'What do you mean you're not going to take it? You never listen to anyone. That's your problem. If the doctor says you should be on it, then you should be on it.' "

Karen's erratic cycle was a clue to the fact that she was in fact dealing with symptoms caused by fluctuating levels of estrogen with no progesterone to balance it. Unfortunately, many people assume that symptoms like forgetfulness and tiredness or an early, a missing, or late period are psychological in nature.

It's important to keep track of any symptoms you might be experiencing. You should note when symptoms occur, the intensity, and anything else that can help you describe their nature. This provides your doctor with a picture of when the symptoms are occurring in relation to the menses. Which symptoms appear to be related to the cycle and which appear to happen at all times?

It's important to ask your doctor questions, even those you might feel are pretty basic. I have many patients who get flustered during their annual exams. Some now hand me a sheet of questions. These are questions they might forget to ask or end up feeling it's stupid to ask, but once it's all down on paper, we can go through them one by one.

## Questions Women Ask

### *How do I know if I've ovulated?*

There are women who seem to know when they ovulate, and there are women who have no clue.

Regular, cyclic menses is the hallmark of ovulation. There are thirteen lunar months in a calendar year, so if you get a menses every twenty-eight days, that will be thirteen cycles in a calendar year.

In addition to regular, cyclic menses, a very predictable premenstrual pattern of symptoms, or what I think of as a premenstrual "aura," indicates ovulation. Whether it be craving chocolate or getting a pimple or bloating or whatever, it's predictable.

The hallmark of anovulatory cycles is their unpredictability. They vary in terms of menstrual flow and also in terms of the presence or absence of premenstrual symptoms.

If you really want to know if you've ovulated, ultrasound can pinpoint ovulation by showing the presence of a corpus luteum in the ovary and secretory endometrium in the uterus — both indicative of ovulation. Or, if your cycle is normally twenty-seven to twenty-nine days, a blood test for progesterone done around day twenty-two, twenty-three, or twenty-four is 100 percent reliable. If you have ovulated there will be progesterone in your blood. If you have not, there will be none.

Some women rely on basal body temperature to tell if they have ovulated. (The production of progesterone with ovulation causes a temperature elevation of about a degree.) I find this to be highly unreliable and cumbersome. Other women use their cervical mucus as a clue. (This is long and stringy right before ovulation – the medical term is *spinbarkeit* — and then changes abruptly to watery mucus with ovulation.) This is helpful for some, but most of my patients find it's not of great reliability.

*How is what I'm experiencing different from being in menopause?*
In menopause your body makes no estrogen and no progesterone, and menstruation stops. This does not occur suddenly, like turning off a faucet. It's gradual. The immediate forerunner of menopause is a set of symptoms that are *not* usually subtle, such as a dry vagina and hot flashes. These symptoms are caused by very low levels of estrogen as well as rising levels of FSH (follicle stimulating hormone).

Women who are entering perimenopause are generally still making estrogen, although the levels may fluctuate. The distinction is important. If a doctor misreads the signs and gives estrogen supplements to a woman whose problems are caused by unopposed estrogen, the symptoms may be compounded.

***How exactly does a doctor determine that a woman's symptoms are
due to unopposed estrogen instead of something else?***
First a doctor looks at menstrual history, which is why it is so important for women to keep a good calendar. In addition, the doctor inquires about subtle symptoms such as mood changes (depression), free-floating anxiety, sleep disturbances, forgetfulness, changes in libido, difficulty concentrating, etc.

Doctors can also do blood tests to verify this transition. One test measures the level of estradiol in the blood. Estrogen isn't really one hormone but three — estrone, estradiol, and estriol. Estradiol is the predominant estrogen in terms of potency. Estradiol comes mainly from the ovaries, which is why this is the type of estrogen your gynecologist is most interested in.

The second test is for FSH (follicle stimulating hormone) level. FSH is the hormone that tells the ovary to release an egg. It will also appear in your blood.

Sometimes, however, these blood tests can give confusing results. Many patients have estrogen levels that are not in a menopausal range (in other words, they are still making estrogen), but their FSH levels will have started to rise (greater than 30, which is typical for postmenopausal women), and their interpretation when given the laboratory's norms will be in the menopausal status. It appears paradoxical, because the patient's estrogen level is premenopausal and the patient's FSH is postmenopausal.

How does this happen? Recall that the pituitary makes FSH. As the follicles respond by producing estrogen, there is feedback to the pituitary that signals it to stop producing FSH. In menopause, because there are no follicles in the ovaries that are responding and therefore no estrogen production, the pituitary continues to make more and more FSH, while the ovaries continue to be unresponsive. In perimenopause, however, sometimes an ovary responds and sometimes it doesn't. Sometimes it responds only given a high level of FSH.

The ovaries do not turn themselves off like a light switch. They often "sputter." I have seen numerous women whose readings were in a menopausal range, and then they subsequently had a last gasp of ovarian function, produced some estrogen, had some bleeding, and a new measurement showed them to be in a nonmenopausal range. However, this clearly is near the end of transition.

What this means to you is that a single measurement of FSH or estradiol may be insufficient in telling you whether you're perimenopausal or menopausal. It also means you'd be wise to request both an FSH test and a test for estradiol in your blood and repeat these tests more than once if your fertility is an issue or if you've been told that you're in menopause. If a doctor measures only estradiol, he or she may conclude that you are not menopausal if you still make some estrogen. If FSH is the only thing tested, and the reading is high, a doctor might conclude that you are menopausal and recommend hormone replacement therapy when in fact it isn't necessary yet. (I discuss hormone replacement therapy at length in chapter 11.)

Any diagnosis I make is aided greatly by the use of transvaginal ultrasound as part of the overall pelvic exam. You can ask for this test. What does this simple office procedure show? If a patient is indeed having episodes of anovulation and unopposed estrogen, the doctor expects to see a nonsecretory endometrium and not to find a corpus luteum in either ovary on ultrasound. He or she expects to see multiple follicles present and a relatively homogenous uterine lining suggestive of unopposed estrogen.

### Can I be thirty-one and going into perimenopause?
The medical field defines menopause (not perimenopause) as the cessation of menses for at least six months due to a depletion of ovarian

follicles. We further know that the national average age for menopause is 51.4 years. What I am referring to as perimenopause, in my experience, can occupy a short time span or up to a whole decade. If someone has actual menopause at forty-six or forty-seven (which is not uncommon), her perimenopause conceivably can start in the midthirties.

We have no great measure of perimenopausal status. Like all things in medicine, there is a range that is defined by a bell-shaped curve. Think of a variable like height. If I took 10,000 women and grouped them by height, their numbers would follow a bell-shaped curve. Most would be 5'4", 5'5", 5'3", but some would be 4'11" and some would be 6'2".

There is a similar range or bell-shaped curve for perimenopausal symptoms and years of their occurrence. Most women will fall somewhere in the middle, but it's also possible to be at one of the two extremes. A woman in her early to midthirties might have such symptomatology the way some women are 4'11" or 6'2".

*Can I get pregnant if I'm in perimenopause?*
Absolutely. When you are still ovulating, whether that's once every month or once every six months, you can become pregnant.

*Is there anything a woman can do to delay the onset of perimenopause? My mother and sister went through menopause in their forties.*
It is impossible to say how much of perimenopause/menopause is genetic. Certainly when a woman tells me that her mother and both of her older sisters went through their "changes" in their early forties, I understand why she thinks she will as well.

I tell my patients that genes are incredibly powerful. Although menopause is not like blue eyes (if your mother and father both have blue eyes, you will definitely have blue eyes), one should never underestimate its hereditary component. However, having said that, I think there is no question that most things have a genetic predisposition and then need environmental influences to cause their expression.

Some of the other factors that seem to be good predictors that a woman will reach menopause slightly younger than her peers include:

- Smoking cigarettes, especially more than half a pack a day
- Being more than ten pounds underweight
- Having had surgery to remove all or part of an ovary
- Having been treated for cancer with chemotherapy or abdominal-radiation therapy

*Is there any way to make hormones without drugs, by exercising, for example?*

No, there is no way to make hormones. It is likely that your experience in the transition, depending on your endogenous hormone levels, will be that much easier if you have a positive outlook, if you are exercising regularly, and if you have made healthy lifestyle choices. But these choices do not make hormones.

*Is it true that it is inevitable that you will gain fifteen pounds in the decade before menopause?*

Absolutely not. Many women lose weight in perimenopause. Still, there are many women whose metabolisms do change as they get older and who find they cannot eat the same amount they used to and maintain the same proportions and weight.

*I've been having trouble sleeping lately, and I can't concentrate at work the way I used to. But I'm also under a lot of stress since my father became ill. How do I know if what I'm experiencing is related to perimenopause or stress?*

It isn't necessarily an either/or situation. What I do in cases like this is to provide hormonal treatment for perimenopause symptoms in the form of *cycle regulators* — I discuss the exact nature of this treatment in chapter 3. Hormonal treatment can remove whatever component of your symptoms is hormonally mediated. The more improvement, the more the problem was caused by your hormones.

*Why does it hurt when I ovulate? I can always tell when it's happening because I get a pain on one side or the other every month.*

When you ovulate there is usually a dominant follicle that bursts and produces an egg. The bursting of the follicle capsule to release the egg and the fluid surrounding the egg is one cause of the pain. The Germans named the pain *Mittleschmerz.*

The small amount of fluid that is released from a normal-size dominant follicle (2.5 cm) acts as an irritant to the pelvic peritoneum, and it can cause soreness and pain as well.

*I'm forty-seven and I'm not experiencing any symptoms. How likely
am I to be one of the lucky ones?*

The median age of the onset of perimenopause is 47.5 years, although it can start earlier or later. As many as 70 percent of women in their forties experience a change in their menstrual cycles. About 35 percent of women experience their first episodes of depression during perimenopause. Twenty to forty percent complain of sleep problems. Up to 50 percent ultimately experience hot flashes as they get close to actual menopause. And yes, there are women who experience nothing at all. There are also women who do not attribute these symptoms to their changing patterns of ovulation and never seek medical intervention or even tell their medical doctors about what they're experiencing psychologically. All in all, there are many women who avoid the roller coaster of transition or whose symptoms are very mild.

*I've always figured that menopause is something you can't do
anything about, so why worry about it until it happens?*

You can shape the course of it more than you think. It will depend on what you do in the decade before it. Consider the philosophy most women use when they think about retirement. It may not be something that will happen for years, but you learn about IRAs and 401Ks now because you're savvy enough to want a plan. You prepare for it now to make it easier later. No crisis. No regrets. It's the same with the decade before menopause.

Patients who learn about hormones and their monthly cycles now can take the steps necessary to put an end to a host of annoying symptoms that can occur at this time. And they can begin to make lifestyle changes that will reap benefits in years to come.

# 2

# A CLOSER LOOK AT YOUR SYMPTOMS

It's estimated that 10 percent of perimenopausal women don't experience any symptoms at all. They just eventually stop having their periods. That leaves 90 percent of women who are going to enter transition and experience symptoms they've never had before. These women want to know, *Is this serious? Should I call my doctor? Is this perimenopause or something else entirely?*

This chapter will help you recognize what symptoms you can expect from a shifting hormonal cycle and when you should look further than perimenopause for the cause.

## Didn't I Just Have My Period Last Week?

There are essentially two types of perimenopausal symptoms. On the one hand are the bleeding symptoms. On the other hand there are psychological symptoms. Let's look at the changes that occur in the menstrual cycle first.

Doctors used to say that abnormal bleeding was too heavy, too little, or at the wrong time of the month. But the more we learn about the decade before menopause, the more this definition has to stretch. I've already mentioned that in terms of bleeding, "abnormal" amounts can be very typical during perimenopause. Yet there is such a range of changing patterns that it helps to understand the variations that can occur. Your bleeding pattern may seem so bizarre at times that you can't imagine that other women go through this, but I assure you they do.

The most frequent reported menstrual changes during peri-menopause include the following:

- Your period may go on and on. It used to last three days; now it's five, six, or more. Some women report having periods three weeks of the month.
- Your period may disappear for several months.
- A once-regular cycle goes awry. You can no longer plan vacations or other events around your period because you're no longer sure when it will come. You flow, you spot, you stop. Then, in the middle of the annual corporate meeting, a deluge.
- You may have your first experience with very heavy bleeding.
- You may begin to have your period twice a month.

All of these changes can be comprehended, if not predicted, once you understand what's happening to your body. What follows are the experiences of several of my patients, which may help you further understand your own changes.

## The Missing Period

"To be honest, I'm not the most careful diaphragm user," Anita, forty-two, admitted. "I use it every time, but sometimes I'm out of gel and I think, *'So what? The diaphragm itself will probably do the trick.'* My friends in their forties are having a terrible time getting pregnant. I guess I got sloppy with the whole procedure, thinking it can't happen to me."

Thus, Anita's first thought when she missed her period was "Oh, no!" She went immediately to the drugstore to buy an over-the-counter pregnancy test. "The test was negative. I tested myself again the next day with the same result.

"I got the sugar cravings and breast tenderness like any other month, but no period. I spent about sixty dollars on pregnancy tests, using different brands, when my sister said, 'For goodness sake, it will be cheaper to just go to the doctor.' "

WHAT TO RULE OUT: A missing period is scary but often normal at this stage. The obvious thing every woman needs to rule out when she misses her period is pregnancy. Over-the-counter pregnancy tests can give you a valid reading often from the first day your period is late. They work by picking up signs of hormones in your blood that are only present during pregnancy. Because many women confuse the dates of their menstrual cycles, if your pregnancy test result is negative and your period still doesn't come in another week, take a second test. The tests are often sold in pairs for this purpose.

Suppose you aren't pregnant. The hormones responsible for menstruation can also be disrupted by emotional factors, such as the stress of a divorce, a new job, or a death in the family. Consider the stresses in your life over the past couple of months. Is there anything unusual?

Positive events can also cause stress. Getting married, buying a home, or getting a promotion at work are experiences that can be thrilling, but they can also disrupt the menstrual cycle due to the added stress.

Women who go off oral contraceptive pills frequently find that it takes several months for their cycles to become regular again. You should start having regular periods within three months of stopping birth-control pills, but this doesn't occur for every woman. Progesterone, which I talk about at length in the next chapter, can help you get back on track and keep your uterine lining from being overstimulated.

IS IT PERIMENOPAUSE? Overall, it is very common to miss your period at the time of perimenopause. This is often the first sign of anovulation. Missing a period is not dangerous to you and is nothing to be alarmed about. Have you been having symptoms that usually signal the beginning of your period, such as tender breasts or bloating or acne? If you have, and these then went away, it's possible that your hormone levels were not enough in synch during your cycle to cause ovulation, or they may have fallen off somewhere in the middle of the cycle. If no follicle develops, the uterine lining does not thicken and is not sloughed off. Therefore you get no period. If you do not ovulate and make progesterone, and the estrogen level stays relatively constant, the lining will thicken but won't slough off. So, no period as well.

In any case, there are tests your doctor can perform, notably a test for progesterone, to see if you've ovulated. An ultrasound exam at the right time of the month can give you absolute assurance, and I discuss why this is so useful in chapter 7.

## The Period That Disappears for Months

At forty-five, Jayne went three months without a period. "I knew I wasn't pregnant. I didn't have a sexual partner. There was just a sudden dawning that my period hadn't come in a while. I tried to reconstruct the date of my last period, and I really couldn't.

"When a month went by from the day I first noticed I was late, I knew I wasn't imagining this. My best friend said, 'Don't you remember? You had your period at Kevin's [her son's] birthday party. You took my last tampon, and I could have clobbered you a week later when I got mine.'"

When Jayne did the math, she realized Kevin's party had been three months earlier. That brought her to the doctor. Her biggest concern was that she never felt premenstrual; it was as if her period had just vanished. "Is this menopause at forty-five? It seems too soon."

WHAT TO RULE OUT: Jayne knew she wasn't pregnant. Jayne was only forty-five, but it is not unusual for a woman to reach menopause at that age. Tracking other symptoms that occur at this time is helpful. For instance, are you experiencing a vagina that seems drier than normal? Have you noticed that you are waking up perspiring heavily during the night? Are you enduring profuse sweating, weakness, or faintness during the day? These are signs of estrogen depletion. However, a woman's period can be quite erratic when she is still making estrogen and not nearly as close to menopause as she thinks.

Disorders of the pituitary gland are a common reason for a period that disappears for months in women who are not in menopause. An underactive or overactive thyroid gland, known respectively as hypothyroidism and hyperthyroidism, can be the culprit. A simple blood test can tell you if you are suffering from either of these. Also, excess prolactin, a pituitary hormone that stimulates breast milk production, can cause a lack of menses. This is often associated with discharge from the nipple. It is also diagnosed with a blood test.

There are other, less frequent reasons women can stop having their menstrual cycles. Very heavy drinkers can develop cirrhosis of the liver, and their menstrual cycles will stop. Generally this will not be the first sign of such a disorder. You will have experienced jaundice, gastrointestinal problems, a distended stomach from fluid retention, and an allover ill feeling.

Dilatation and curettage (D&C) that hasn't healed properly and left scar tissue can also cause a loss of your period. A pelvic exam can rule out ovarian cysts or other growths than can cause you to skip your period.

Exercise, while generally helpful to you, can cause menstruation to come to a halt if you go at it in a way that's extreme. Let me give an example. A patient of mine, Alicia, was sent to cover the Tour de France for a major magazine. After spending weeks with the young cyclists, she came home enamored with the whole idea of long-distance biking. At thirty-six, she was twenty-five pounds overweight, and she saw this as a way to begin a weight-loss program she could stick with.

She joined cycling clubs, where she met other women who were serious about the sport. They encouraged her to train for a race that was being held that fall. She began riding an hour and a half every day. She lost weight rapidly.

Excited by the distances she was becoming capable of, she went on the club's biking trips on weekends. Sometimes those weekend trips covered fifty to a hundred miles or more. She rode with bikers who had been riding much longer than she, and she often ended up walking her bike for miles, or riding up the hills in the truck that always accompanied the bikers. This was embarrassing and she would dedicate herself to doing better the next weekend.

She went at her training so hard in a space of three months that she stopped having her period, because her body fat was reduced dramatically and replaced by muscle. She went for four months without a period, until an injury forced her to stop cycling.

There are many women who get into exercise with a vengeance for the first time in their thirties or forties. Perhaps it's the discovery of a new spinning class, or a particularly fun aerobics teacher, or the sudden desire to see if at this point in life one is still fit enough to run a marathon. This new regime is stressful to the body. Once your body fat level dips too low, there's a good chance your period will stop. Your body is no longer producing enough estrogen for ovulation to occur.

A rapid weight loss for other reasons, mainly fad diets, can also cause your period to stop. So can a large weight gain. Fifteen pounds may not do it, but extreme weight change can. Weight gain can also raise insulin levels, which can stimulate the body to produce androgens, hormones that produce male or masculine characteristics.

It's particularly important to seek treatment if you have gone without your period for six months when you aren't pregnant, lactating, or in menopause. You want to guard against possible bone loss (from low estrogen) and overstimulation of the endometrial lining (from high estrogen), which is one cause of endometrial cancer. Hormone therapy is often recommended for athletes who find themselves in this situation.

IS IT PERIMENOPAUSE? Nine times out of ten, if you are between the ages of thirty-five and fifty, the answer to your missing period is perimenopause. A missing period for several months could be signaling menopause. An FSH test and a test for estrogen will give you those answers.

## The Period That Seems as if It Will Never Stop

"I'm not exaggerating when I tell you that my period lasted for more than two weeks," Diane, forty, explained, exasperated. "I was sick of all of this bleeding. I kept waiting for the last day, and there was never a last day."

WHAT TO RULE OUT: Is it a period, or is it midcycle spotting? It's important to keep track of how much bleeding there is. How heavy is it? Some women use menstrual calendars, where they designate each day as light, moderate, or heavy.

What kind of birth control are you using? An IUD can be the cause of a longer than average bleeding cycle. Is there any possibility of a miscarriage?

Ongoing bleeding could be due to a polyp. Pelvic infection, especially if your abdomen hurts and you have a fever or vaginal discharge, is another possibility. And it must be ascertained that the bleeding is coming from the vagina, not the rectum or bladder.

Diabetes, thyroid problems, and kidney disease should always be ruled out as causes of a normal menstrual cycle that suddenly goes awry.

Age is important. If you're over fifty, and a period that never stops comes after a year or so of not menstruating, it goes by the term "postmenopausal bleeding." In this scenario, contact with a gynecologist is mandatory. Such bleeding must be investigated. I and many other doctors are using ultrasound and fluid-enhanced ultrasound instead of biopsy or D&C to rule out hyperplasia, which I discuss at length in chapter 7.

**IS IT PERIMENOPAUSE?** It's the most frequent diagnosis for bleeding that goes on longer than usual in a woman age thirty-five to fifty, but blood tests, a Pap test, and a sonogram would be the first steps in determining this. See your doctor.

## The Period That Comes Twice a Month

"Sure, I've been regular for the last six months," Meghan, forty-two, assured me. "Twice a month, like clockwork."

There is nothing more galling for most women than to find that they are having two periods each month. Why does this happen?

**WHAT TO RULE OUT:** Are you really having your period every twenty-one days or so, which can be normal, or are you having midcycle spotting? The character of your flow is important. Is it the same as usual, or heavy at one point in the month and much lighter later, which would signal spotting? Spotting between cycles can be a part of normal ovulation. However, you want to rule out endometrial cancer, hyperplasia, and polyps, which are also causes of midcycle spotting. Never diagnose midcycle spotting or spotting that occurs after sexual intercourse yourself. Call your doctor.

**IS IT PERIMENOPAUSE?** As women age, their menstrual cycles become shorter because they ovulate earlier. A woman's cycle can shorten to as little as twenty days during perimenopause, which would give you a period once every three weeks, and this can be entirely normal. If your flow isn't excessive, what you're experiencing can be normal for you, but on a tighter schedule. The phase of your cycle when the follicle grows and then bursts is now less than fourteen days. You ovulate, but your cycle is shorter.

## The Heavy Period

Janice's periods got so heavy she could no longer wear tampons because she had to change them so frequently. "It was very scary because the blood was so clotty. I thought I had been pregnant and I was having a miscarriage. I felt tired and dizzy much of the time. The bleeding was making it difficult to leave the house."

**WHAT TO RULE OUT:** Miscarriage is the first thing to rule out when one experiences an unusually heavy, clotty bleed. But heavy or prolonged bleeding is very common, and it can come from a host of causes. Fibroid tumors are one cause. Pelvic infection or an IUD that's gone awry are also reasons for heavy bleeding. Does your lower abdomen hurt? Did the pain come on slowly, and do you have a fever and discharge from your vagina?

It is also true that you can have abnormal bleeding — either heavy or at the wrong time or both — from cancer, hyperplasia, or polyps. Endometriosis, a disease in which the tissue from the lining of the uterus grows in other areas in the pelvis, is a very common cause of heavy and painful bleeding.

A dysfunction of the hypothalamus, pituitary, or adrenal glands can cause heavy bleeding. So can thyroid problems.

In contemporary gynecology, heavy bleeding is known as "menorrhagia," or uterine bleeding characterized by excessive flow or long duration. It is defined as more than 80 cc (5 tablespoons) in a period or more than the regular number of days. The trouble is, what's normal for one woman may be excessive for another, and women aren't measuring menses in a test tube.

If your menses can be dealt with by a super-plus tampon, it's probably within a normal range.

If you have always had three-day periods where you never bled through a sanitary pad or a tampon, and all of a sudden the last two have lasted seven days and you've ruined three pairs of pants, this is abnormal for you.

IS IT PERIMENOPAUSE? You can have very heavy, very frightening bleeding from nothing more than a hormonal imbalance. In fact, this is true for more than 75 percent of women who experience heavy bleeding episodes in their thirties and forties. The estrogen you are making stimulates the uterine lining to build up. It thickens. You don't ovulate, and estrogen continues to stimulate the growth of the endometrium. The lining gets thicker and thicker with no progesterone to trigger its release. Then the endometrium is destabilized, and your blood flow is heavy as it releases a larger than average lining. The result can be heavy, clotty bleeding that is different from the menstrual periods you've experienced before.

Avoid hot baths if you are bleeding heavily. The heat dilates blood vessels, increasing your flow. Aspirin can also lower the ability of platelets to clot, exacerbating your bleeding. Try a nonaspirin pain reliever if you are having cramps.

## A Cycle That's Suddenly Way Off

"For years, I could almost set my watch by my period," says Laura, forty-four. "Not only did it arrive every twenty-seven days, but always in the morning. I'd get a breakout the week before, also on schedule. My period was heavy the first day, with a lot of cramps. But it was lighter on the second, lightest on the third, and then gone on the fourth day. My friends thought I was the luckiest person in the world to be that regular.

"At thirty-seven, the pattern changed. My period came on time. But it was light. I'd almost call it spotting. Then it came full force for one day. Then it stopped for three days. Then it came heavily for three more days. I ended up in bed, feeling absolutely sick and exhausted. My first thought was did I have some kind of blockage, so my period couldn't get out at first? I didn't know what to think.

"It was more of the same the next month. I'd think when I hadn't bled for two days, 'Am I through with this? Dare I wear my white slacks?' Feeling safe, I'd go to sleep without a tampon and wake up with ruined sheets. I started just using tampons every day because I never knew whether I'd have my period or not. But the tampons hurt on days when I didn't bleed, especially when I went to remove them."

**WHAT TO RULE OUT:** If you've just started on the Pill, your bleeding can be erratic at first. Antidepressants and tranquilizers in rare cases cause irregular periods, as they can interfere with the brain's ovulation signals.

**IS IT PERIMENOPAUSE?** Fluctuating levels of unopposed estrogen can indeed cause irregular shedding of the endometrium. This lining is not sloughed off evenly at just one time because of the shifting nature of your hormones. Therefore, you get heavy one day, light the next, heavy again the day after, and so on as the lining sloughs off gradually.

## The Very Light Period

"I wouldn't call the period I had last month a period. It was more like spotting. I kept thinking, 'Okay, let's get on with it.' I had my period pretty much on schedule, but still, I felt like I didn't really have it. Is very light bleeding dangerous?"

**WHAT TO RULE OUT:** The various possibilities include pregnancy, birth-control pills, and menopause. You should also consider how active you are physically and if your general health has changed. Crushing exercise programs and unwise diet practices such as fasting have stopped many women from having regular ovulatory cycles, regardless of their age. An underactive thyroid gland can also be the culprit.

Light bleeding at abnormal times can be caused by injury to the vagina (vigorous intercourse or masturbation compounded by vaginal dryness), herpes sores, stopping or starting estrogen therapy, low thyroid function, or an IUD.

The most important thing to figure out is whether the bleeding is spotting between periods or your period. Keeping a good calendar will give you peace of mind.

IS IT PERIMENOPAUSE? If you don't produce as much estrogen, your uterine lining will be thin. When you get your period, it will be lighter. Even with ovulation, as some women age the flow can get lighter.

## When Should You Call Your Doctor About Bleeding?

Any bleeding that worries you is enough to signal a call to your doctor. These can be very normal signs of perimenopause, but you should always discuss the following changes in your cycle with your doctor to rule out other causes:

- A very heavy period with clots
- Spotting or bleeding between periods
- Bleeding after sex
- Unusually severe cramps — more intense than you've ever experienced
- Bleeding when you haven't had a period for more than twelve months

## Other Physical Symptoms and What They Mean

### Killer Cramps

Shooting pains in your abdomen may remind you of the days when you were fifteen and first experiencing your period. You remember rolling up in a ball in your bedroom, praying for the cramps to pass, and they did. But that was teenage stuff. Why are these crushing cramps back suddenly?

WHAT TO RULE OUT: Some common causes of pelvic pain are fibroids and scarring left by sexually transmitted diseases, notably pelvic inflammatory disease. Endometriosis — when uterine tissue appears elsewhere in the pelvis and bleeds or swells as it reacts to your cycle of hormones — can also cause severe pain.

IS IT PERIMENOPAUSE? The medical term for painful cramps is "dysmenorrhea," and more than half of menstruating women suffer from it. What causes it? Most likely, prostaglandins. Prostaglandins are released from the endometrium right before your period. They produce uterine contractions, and these can be painful. The contractions are often accompanied by nausea and diarrhea. Call your doctor if the pain is unusually intense, or if it is accompanied by fever, which could signal an infection. Your doctor can help you assess whether your cramps are due to perimenopause or something else.

### Breast Soreness

Chances are if you're like most women, you experience discomfort in your breasts the week before your period. Estrogen stimulates the growth of milk glands and ducts. Progesterone can cause fluid retention, which creates tension in the breasts.

WHAT TO RULE OUT: Sometimes a woman's breasts can be painful fifteen days out of every month. However, be alert to the fact that if your breasts begin to really ache badly or feel hard and tender, you may be experiencing an attack of mastalgia. While doctors do not know what causes mastalgia, it is theorized that it is caused by the breasts' sensitivity to changing hormones at perimenopause, because it generally occurs in women over forty.

Although any breast soreness can be uncomfortable, it is not uncommon for a woman having an attack of mastalgia to feel pain in the nipple and not want anything to touch her breasts. Mastalgia can be scary for women who think "breast cancer" when they experience their first attack. However, pain is not usually cited as a symptom of breast cancer. Breast cancer is usually signaled by symptoms such as lumps in or near your breast, changes in the size of your breast, a discharge from your nipple, dimpled skin, or an inverted nipple, none of which causes pain.

A special note about nipple discharge. Women have tiny structures that look like whiteheads around the nipples. If you squeeze them, a fluid will come out, sometimes hardened and yellow. This is not the same as nipple discharge. These structures come from the oil that lubricates the nipple. They can become clogged, just as the pores that lubricate your face with oil can become clogged and form whiteheads.

IS IT PERIMENOPAUSE? Research has not unveiled any direct link between perimenopause and increased breast pain, but bloated, painful breasts are a complaint of many women during their menstrual cycles. In any case, any breast pain that is suddenly more severe than what is normal for you should be discussed with your doctor, who may want to examine your breasts.

## Symptoms That Aren't All in Your Head: What They Are and How to Recognize Them

### Forgetfulness: "I came into this room for something. . . . Now what was it?"

Aurora, forty-six, says, "I was taking my daughter to the pediatrician. He had moved to a new office building, so I had to look up his name on the directory. I blanked on the name. I couldn't even remember what letter it started with. So here I was in the lobby, feeling totally lost, turning to my three-year-old and saying, 'Honey, you know that nice doctor who gave you those stickers last time? Do you remember his name?' "

WHAT TO RULE OUT: Is it anxiety? Nervousness is one reason people have bouts of forgetfulness, as when you suddenly forget everything you wanted to say because you're so anxious when you're called upon to speak to a group. There are many triggers for anxiety, and in Aurora's case, taking her daughter to the pediatrician could well be one of them.

Be aware that many tranquilizers, including Valium or Xanax, and sleeping pills such as Halcion and Restoril have side effects that include loss of memory.

If you're confused as well as forgetful, doctors will rule out brain tumors, head injuries, and very poor nutrition. These diagnoses are very rare for a woman your age, and I include them not to scare you but to alert you to the fact that I know many women who have been to the neurologist, the psychiatrist, and the allergist before they finally reach the gynecologist.

Probably nothing is so irritating to a woman balancing a challenging schedule than to feel as if her memory is failing. Although it's natural for our ability to retrieve information to slow down with age, it's unlikely that an otherwise healthy woman in her forties who can't remember what she drove to the sporting-goods store for is experiencing premature dementia.

IS IT PERIMENOPAUSE? Forgetfulness is one of the most frequent complaints women have when their menstrual cycles first go awry, but they don't always make the connection. The symptom can occur years before you stop having your period. Medical science has yet to determine why fluctuating levels of unopposed estrogen tend to cause women to have trouble with short-term memory. Scientists know that the hippocampus, the part of the brain associated with memory, is loaded with estrogen receptors. It is theorized that as estrogen levels begin to decrease, or to spike and drop, the brain cannot retrieve information as well.

These episodes can be frightening. Not being able to spell familiar words or to finish a train of thought can make you feel as if your mind is going. The incidents of forgetfulness can be bizarre. One woman told me she could not recall her brother's name for half an hour and was terrified.

Bringing your menstrual calendar into your doctor's office and having a frank discussion about your general health, nutrition, and stress level can help you begin to determine if your bouts of forgetfulness are the beginning of perimenopause. If they are, realize you're not developing Alzheimer's disease. Your estrogen levels aren't going to cause amnesia. But you may experience a lot of tip-of-the-tongue naming trouble. And you are certainly in the normal range if you find that you need to make lists to remember what groceries you need, if phone numbers and names are difficult to retrieve, if you walk into a room and forget what you went there to get, and if trying to memorize a long list of just about anything becomes difficult and irritating.

## Difficulty Concentrating: "I think I read this page before."

You're feeling unfocused. You used to make it a point to read every book you bought from cover to cover, and now you have no patience even to read a magazine article. Your friend has to give you directions to the restaurant five times — you just can't seem to focus.

WHAT TO RULE OUT: Generally, difficulty concentrating is attributed to the stresses of midlife. If you're having trouble sleeping, you may find yourself spacy the next day. What about those drugs in your medicine cabinet? Antihistamines and many allergy pills can cause difficulty concentrating.

IS IT PERIMENOPAUSE? Medical science has not specifically proven what the link is between estrogen and concentration or other cognitive abilities, but women who receive HRT report that their ability to concentrate improves. Low estrogen levels affect the ability to learn new facts and skills. Fluctuating levels of unopposed estrogen have also been linked to difficulty concentrating.

## Mood Swings: "I was feeling fine a minute ago."

It's a very lucky woman who doesn't know about premenstrual moodiness, because she's never experienced it. But now it seems to happen at all times of the month.

I want to emphasize that women at this stage in their lives do not come into my office telling me that they are "cracking up," or "freaking out," or going crazy. They don't fit old stereotypes about women with raging hormones, incapacitated and on the brink.

It is much more subtle. Women talk about heightened sensitivity. Of being irritable. Of experiencing more than the usual PMS moodiness. Of doing what they've always done but without the same enthusiasm. One woman described it as being like having a virus that concerned her only because it didn't go away in a few days.

Are you suddenly quick to anger? You're not alone. As one woman tells it, "I was riding my bike home after a day in the park, and I made a right turn onto my block. There were a couple of guys, maybe in their twenties, in a convertible behind me, trying to turn right onto the same block. I swung too far out for their taste, I guess. The guy honked at me and yelled. 'Why don't you learn how to ride a bike?'

" 'Why don't you learn to drive a car?' I shouted back. Did they think they owned the road?

"He screamed an insult. I screamed back a bigger insult about his car. This was totally unlike me, but I was angry. He slammed on his brakes. My husband, a half a block ahead of me, pedaled back double speed, waving the guys off. He grabbed my arm and said, 'What are you doing? You want to have a screaming match with strangers? People get shot for less. This is the city, you know.' I didn't care. This seemed like such a tremendous issue all of a sudden. 'Why should I have to take any shit from some loser in a cheap convertible?'

"Two minutes later I felt like a fool. My husband looked at me like he was really worried about me."

There's a joke that comes up in many books about menopause: "I'm out of estrogen, and I have a gun." It's theorized that estrogen affects neurotransmitters like serotonin and dopamine in the brain, which help regulate emotions.

In any case, being quick to anger is a symptom many of my patients report along with a changing menstrual cycle.

**WHAT TO RULE OUT:** Clinical depression and anxiety need to be ruled out. But realize you can have depression and anxiety secondary to a changing hormonal balance. Certain drugs for allergies and some over-the-counter cold medicines have been known to cause anxiety as well. Fad diet pills are largely caffeine; they can make you irritable one moment and listless the next.

**IS IT PERIMENOPAUSE?** Progesterone is usually the culprit when women complain of moodiness. It tends to bring on negative moods. Estrogen has a tranquilizing effect. When your estrogen levels are ebbing, moodiness can result.

### Headaches: "Is this a brain tumor?"

"The night before my period, I get a headache on one side," explains Mara, thirty-eight. "It lasts all the next day. It happens every month, right on schedule, but only for a day. Suddenly, though, it seems like I'm having this headache every other week. When I'm stressed or I've had too much to drink, I get headaches. If I try to read in a car, I get an instant, booming headache. But getting these headaches for no reason is starting to get scary. I worry that it could be a brain tumor or something very serious."

Many women are used to experiencing headaches right before their periods begin, but in perimenopause the rise and fall of estrogen levels can cause headaches to become more frequent. Women may complain of a different kind of headache that starts for no apparent reason and won't go away with the usual remedies like rest or aspirin.

**WHAT TO RULE OUT:** There are many, many things that can cause headaches. Eyestrain, medications, glaucoma, sinus problems, hunger, low blood sugar, toothaches, high blood pressure, and head injuries are just some of the possibilities. You should always discuss a severe headache with a physician.

**IS IT PERIMENOPAUSE?** Be reassured that 90 percent of headaches are due to tension and migraine. The most common headache is a tension headache. This is an ache, sometimes described as a tightness or pressure, usually felt in the back of the head or neck. People can have tension headaches that continue for months. The biggest factor here isn't hormones but stress.

You may have read that the headache caused by a brain tumor gets severe over time and is frequently accompanied by vomiting. It isn't unreasonable for you to think you have a brain tumor when you first experience a migraine. Migraines can be agonizing.

Premenstrual migraines are common, and they can occur for the first time during perimenopause. It's believed that these headaches are caused by fluctuating levels of estrogen, particularly a drop in estrogen after a period of high levels.

How can you tell if your headache is a migraine? Migraines are usually one-sided headaches. They throb and intensify over a period of time. Many women feel nauseous and vomit in the midst of a migraine. There are signs that a migraine is coming. Women who have them frequently recognize these signs. You may feel suddenly tired or out of sorts. Some women complain that light hurts their eyes or that they have other vision problems, such as a misting over of one eye or loss of peripheral vision. Then comes the headache.

These headaches are hard to bear, and it's not unusual for a person in the midst of one to look pale and sick and to feel completely incapacitated. Migraines usually last several hours, but they can last a day or two.

Cluster headaches are a variant of migraines. Typically, you get an extreme pain on one side of your head, sometimes centered in or around one of your eyes. The pain peaks in five or ten minutes and is usually gone in an hour. Unfortunately, the headache often returns several hours later.

Many women find that they no longer have migraine headaches after menopause. During the transitional period, when premenstrual migraines can be at their peak frequency, it's important to work with your physician to develop a treatment regimen. There are several drugs that are effective with migraines. Since dilation of blood vessels causes the pain of a migraine, drugs that can constrict the blood vessels are often prescribed.

Many of my patients are helped most by eliminating the known nonhormonal triggers of migraines — alcohol, chocolate, and MSG — and taking two aspirin and going to bed the minute they feel the symptoms coming on.

### Insomnia: "I can't remember the last time I had a good night's sleep."

Insomnia generally gets worse as one gets closer to the last period. This is because night sweats — hot flashes that occur when you are sleeping — trouble many women when their bodies stop making estrogen.

While night sweats are a signal that you are close to actual menopause, many women complain about waking up in a sweat years before menopause happens. Or they complain that they wake for no reason in the middle of the night and then can't go back to sleep.

Sleeping poorly is a big complaint for people, regardless of their age. For millions of people, bedtime is an invitation to hours of worry. Small annoyances like a truck driving by or a humidifier turning on interrupt sleep. Then come the worries of the day: Did I pay the gas bill or didn't I?

The age we live in is a blessing and a curse. It provides us with so much information so quickly that our minds are in a perpetual state of motion from the moment we wake up to the moment we go to sleep, which makes relaxing enough to fall asleep difficult. And unfortunately, as we age, most of us have a harder time falling asleep no matter what our patterns were before.

**WHAT TO RULE OUT:** Stimulants, such as the hidden ones in cold medicines, fad diet pills, remedies bought at health-food stores (I had one patient who didn't sleep regularly for a week after trying DHEA), and diet sodas can keep you awake. Alcohol can send you to sleep only to wake up three hours later — for the rest of the night. A sedentary lifestyle and sleeping late can also be culprits.

**IS IT PERIMENOPAUSE?** Insomnia alone is not an indicator of peri-menopause. The stress of having subtle symptoms you've never experienced before can keep you up at night. Insomnia can exacerbate every other symptom of perimenopause, so it's important that if you're having trouble sleeping, you talk to your doctor about it and formulate a plan for improving your sleep. The quality of your sleep is a major part of your sense of well-being.

### Free-Floating Anxiety: "I feel like I'm ten feet above everyone else in the room."

The jitters, an inability to concentrate, a queasy stomach — most of us feel some symptoms of anxiety from time to time in a world that grows more complex and unpredictable by the minute.

For the most part, anxiety is situational. Your heart pounds before you give a speech. You're nauseated when your wedding plans go awry. But what if anxiety overtakes you for no apparent reason? Is this something you have to live with?

**WHAT TO RULE OUT:** To diagnose anxiety, a complete physical is indicated. You need to rule out possible causes of your symptoms including hyperthyroidism, disorders of the brain, hypoglycemia, heavy caffeine use, drug abuse, and alcohol withdrawal.

Could you possibly have a generalized anxiety disorder? What is the difference between having an anxiety disorder and just feeling anxious? According to the American Psychiatric Association's *Diagnostic and Statistical Manual of Mental Disorders (DSM-IV)*, the diagnostic criteria for generalized anxiety disorder include the following:

- Excessive anxiety and worry occurring more days than not for at least six months about a number of events or activities

- Difficulty controlling the worry
- Three or more of the following six symptoms for more days than not for the past six months: restlessness or feeling keyed up or on edge; being easily fatigued; difficulty concentrating; irritability; muscle tension; difficulty falling asleep or restless, unsatisfying sleep

If you can identify, take heart in knowing that thousands of people have these symptoms. It doesn't mean you definitely have generalized anxiety disorder, but it is a "heads up" warning to see your doctor.

IS IT PERIMENOPAUSE? Generally, the type of anxiety experienced due to fluctuating levels of unopposed estrogen is subtle, not intense. With something like anxiety, it is difficult for a doctor to determine if it's due solely to perimenopause. Sometimes the only way the doctor and patient know for sure is if the patient is given medication to regulate hormones (I discuss what works in the next chapter) and the anxiety disappears.

## Depression: "What's the use?"

It took five years for Ellen, forty-nine, to get her line of jewelry into a major chain of department stores. This was a chance to take her business to a new level. She was going to have more money, more freedom. It meant the end to the drudgery of showing her work at art fairs in the summer heat, roasting under an umbrella.

Ellen expected to feel ecstatic. But after a week or two, little had changed. "There's this sense of gloom I can't shake. I just feel flat."

WHAT TO RULE OUT: Your feelings may be more than a passing bad mood if you experience at least four of these symptoms for two weeks or more:

- Low energy or tiredness, even when you get enough sleep
- Sleeping too little or too much
- A change in appetite; you gain or lose a significant amount of weight without dieting
- Little interest or pleasure in all or most of your usual activities

- A depressed mood most of the day; feelings of guilt, worthlessness, or hopelessness
- Difficulty concentrating, making decisions
- Thoughts of death or suicide

These are the symptoms of clinical depression. If you experience these symptoms and nothing seems to alleviate them, it's time to seek professional help.

IS IT PERIMENOPAUSE? Researchers maintain that there is no direct link between depression and perimenopause — or menopause, for that matter. Although I've seen few women who meet the criteria for clinical depression due to perimenopause, I've seen plenty who complain of crying and a "What's the use?" feeling. As one of my patients put it, "I just never get much pleasure out of anything. I think this is just me, the way I am."

There is no question that symptoms like forgetfulness, weight gain, or having a surprise period in the middle of a board meeting could make anyone feel depressed. Added to this are your changing hormone levels. Fluctuating estrogen can result in mood swings. Estrogen deprivation may be the source of feeling down or emotionally flat. Estrogen without progesterone to balance it may result in anxiety, a feeling of being off or not oneself.

## Faintness, Dizziness, and Palpitations: "Am I having a heart attack?"

There's probably nothing more daunting to your sense of being in control than feeling as if you're going to faint. Symptoms like dizziness and palpitations are not usually troubling to women at the beginning of perimenopause. It's when one gets closer to actual menopause and a lack of estrogen that these symptoms occur, generally at the time of a hot flash.

It is wise to discuss any of these symptoms with your doctor immediately, as they can be very upsetting to your peace of mind.

WHAT TO RULE OUT: Rapid breathing from exercise or a sudden scare can bring on a feeling of faintness. An infection of the inner ear will cause dizziness. Drugs for high blood pressure can also cause an unsteady feeling if they bring your blood pressure too low. Low blood sugar is another common cause of these symptoms.

Palpitations sometimes unnerve women so much that they are sure they are having a heart attack. Heart attacks are extremely rare before menopause. They generally don't feel like palpitations, but a pressure and squeezing in your chest.

IS IT PERIMENOPAUSE? If your dizziness and heart palpitations are severe, my hunch would be that your symptoms are either from some other cause or from estrogen depletion — the hallmark of menopause. Many women report having palpitations along with a hot flash. As for a milder dizzy, unsteady feeling, women in perimenopause often do complain of periods of time in which they don't feel like themselves.

## Questions Women Ask

*How do I know I'm having perimenopause symptoms and not just PMS?*

You might be having PMS. Of course, one of the primary symptoms of perimenopause is worse-than-usual PMS. But I have mentioned before that regular menses have a premenstrual aura, whether that's a pimple, a case of cramps, or a craving for chocolate. This happens, and within a week your period arrives. In perimenopause, this can still be the case, but more often, these symptoms seem to come at any time of the month. Or you have a PMS symptom, such as a migraine or water retention, that you've never had before. What's regular during perimenopause is something that is *irregular.*

*I'm forty-five and I have four children. Over the past years my periods have been heavier instead of lighter. Shouldn't it be the other way around?*

Multiple pregnancies enlarge the uterus. (So do fibroids, for that matter.) The normal size of the uterus in someone who has four or five children is double the size of the uterus of a woman who hasn't had any. As the cavity expands, there is more surface area. Therefore, when you get a normal period, you have double the amount of lining built up in your uterus to shed.

*I'm fifty-one and I am spotting every day. Is this normal, like a long, last period?*

Menopause usually isn't like a faucet that drips and then quits. You should see your doctor to determine the cause of your bleeding. This kind of change in menstrual patterns always warrants an examination.

*Can stress really stop a woman from having a period? I was recently in a car accident, and I'm wondering if that has anything to do with why my period is late.*

Let's say that you are on day twenty-five of an ovulatory cycle and you're in an automobile accident where you aren't hurt but terrified and stressed out for days. You will still get your period. If you already ovulated, fourteen days after ovulation, you will get your period.

What stress can do is cause a lack of ovulation. People who don't ovulate may not get a period for months. An example of this was what occurred during World War II in the concentration camps, when women under tremendous stress didn't menstruate. This was partly due to starvation, but undoubtedly stress was a factor, as even women who received extra food lost their menstrual cycles.

So yes, a death in the family, a change in jobs, going from working days to working nights, studying for the bar exam, travel, and other identifiable stress can throw a woman's cycle off. So can thyroid problems or problems in the pituitary gland.

*Why do some women have much worse perimenopausal symptoms than others?*

That's like asking why some women have more difficult labor pains, or more severe menstrual cramps, or why some women are 4'10" and others 5'11". Genetics is probably an issue. Diet, nutrition, and a multitude of factors that we may not understand also contribute to the range of symptomatology you may encounter.

# 3

# YOU DON'T HAVE TO FEEL THIS WAY

Julia, forty-four, was intelligent, athletic, and a dedicated attorney who worked hard but still managed to find time for her passion — horseback riding. Her eight-year-old daughter was becoming an expert rider herself. It was a time in Julia's career and personal life when she couldn't afford two weeks every month of feeling bloated, out of control, moody. But this was exactly what was happening.

The fatigue hit her hard. On her best days, she dragged through her activities feeling just a little off, unlike her natural self. Her temper became short. The active, steady, happy person she used to be began to seem like some other woman. Worse, no one seemed to want to hear about it.

"I'm the oldest in my group of friends," she says. "I could see them rolling their eyes, thinking, Get beyond it. Stop complaining, already. I think I scared them. They didn't want to think that maybe this was something that would happen to them when they hit forty."

Julia had suffered for almost a year when I saw her for the first time. After a pelvic exam and blood tests revealed nothing unusual, I suggested she try low-dose birth-control pills to combat her symptoms. She looked at me, surprised.

"It stopped me in my tracks," she told me later. "Wasn't it going to be dangerous at my age? It seemed odd to go back on the Pill again after all of these years, especially when I didn't have a sexual partner. What about side effects?"

She told me she was uncomfortable about taking birth-control pills. I said, "If I told you that there was a pill that would relieve your symptoms and regulate your hormones — let's call it a *cycle regulator* — would you want to try it?"

She left my office with a prescription for Loestrin 1/20 — a low-dose birth-control pill created specifically for women in their forties. It was a prescription she didn't fill.

Six weeks later I heard from her again. She phoned to ask, "Can I still fill this prescription? I'm yelling at my daughter, fighting with everyone, not sleeping. I can't take this anymore. I'm willing to try anything."

She filled the prescription. Two months later she called to tell me, "I can't believe it. Within three weeks I felt normal again."

But she was calling about her period. It was lighter than she'd had in the past, and she was concerned. I explained that on birth-control pills, the bleeding one has on the week off of medication is not truly a period from a medical point of view. Medically speaking, a period is a menses that occurs two weeks after ovulation. On birth-control pills, no ovulation takes place. What occurs on the week off the medication is referred to as a "withdrawal bleed." This might seem like a small point, but the distinction is important.

I believe that the medical establishment did a great disservice to women by making birth-control pills in twenty-eight-day cycles to mimic the natural cycle. It is somewhat patronizing and confusing to women that the bleed comes every twenty-eight days and that they therefore equate it with their period. When this "period" is not perfectly normal, it frightens them unnecessarily. The bleeding on birth-control pills is totally artificial. The small amounts of estrogen and progesterone in birth-control pills causes a minimal amount of buildup of lining of the endometrial cavity. Whatever small amount of buildup there is is shed in the week of no medication.

Patients often think, "Where has the blood gone?" when there is almost no bleeding. Especially with low-dose pills (20 mcg of estrogen), there is often so little buildup that there is almost no bleeding during the week off medication. This is predictable and desirable.

"Many women think of it as part of the bonus plan," I told Julia as I explained why her bleeding was so light. She began to laugh. "See? I think everything is funny again. I was worried you were going to say I have to go off Loestrin. I never want to go off it and have my hormones do that wacky little dance again. I wish I had done this two years ago."

If the change in Julia after taking low-dose birth-control pills sounds dramatic, it was. I too am sometimes amazed at the effect low-dose birth-control pills have on women whose symptoms have plagued them for years.

## Today's Most Effective Treatment for Perimenopause

Today, low-dose birth-control pills are the most effective treatment for perimenopausal symptoms. True, not all women respond to low-dose birth-control pills as dramatically as Julia did. There are those whose experience is more subtle and others who experience little change at all.

But for many women, the change is dramatic. Hundreds of women have told me, "I can't believe how great I feel. I thought I just had crummy PMS, but now I feel steadier all month long; I wish I had done this years ago."

These are not exactly the kinds of results a woman associates with taking the Pill. One might wonder, "Birth-control pills not to prevent conception but for forgetfulness? A lack of concentration? Moodiness? Depression?"

For a lot of women in the forty-plus age group, the idea of the Pill comes with a lot of baggage. Offer them to a forty-three-year-old woman who has had her tubes tied, and she looks at you like you're crazy. This is why I have begun to refer to these low-dose pills as "cycle regulators."

When I first began prescribing low-dose birth-control pills to older women, it was to help them regulate menstrual cycles that had become erratic. I specialized in this area, so my caseload was skewed in that most of the women I saw experienced problem bleeding. That's when I first began to hear women repeat the same subtle psychological symptoms that compounded their problems — the fatigue, the forgetfulness, the free-floating anxiety, the feeling of not being themselves. Low-dose birth-control pills were equally effective at banishing those symptoms. They regulated their periods, but they also regulated their moods. For Julia, low-dose birth-control pills did what drugs are intended to do — restore health.

## The Pill Has Come a Long Way in Twenty Years

Your decision about whether or not to take low-dose birth-control pills will be easier if you have the right information. Unfortunately, there are still plenty of misconceptions out there.

Let me dispel the myths about oral contraceptives. First of all, you can safely forget the dire warnings from the 1970s about the risks of stroke and heart attack in women over the age of thirty-five taking the Pill. Those studies are now twenty years old — and based on pills that had four to six times more estrogen than they do today. If you are in your forties now, the birth-control pills you may have taken when you were a teenager or in your twenties had either 80 or 50 mcg of estrogen. Today's low-dose pills have about 20.

The requirement for package inserts to contain the warning that oral contraceptives may increase the risk of cardiovascular disease among healthy nonsmoking women over forty was discontinued by the FDA in 1991. This reflects the increased safety of the lower-dose formulations, proven through intensive research studies, as well as the ability to identify many of the factors that put women at risk. I will discuss risk factors later in this chapter.

## How Low-Dose Birth-Control Pills Banish Symptoms of Perimenopause

Birth-control pills consist of combinations of different doses of estrogen and progesterone. They come in packs of twenty-one or twenty-eight. The twenty-eight pack contains seven placebo pills, so a woman continues to take the pills without having to worry about what day it is or losing track of when to start taking them again.

Low-dose birth-control pills work by turning off the ovaries' natural estrogen production and replacing it with a measured amount of estrogen and progesterone all month long. Since it is fluctuating levels of hormones due to anovulatory cycles that are causing the problems in perimenopause, these pills eliminate whatever symptoms may be hormonal. More simply, the Pill gives you the estrogen you need for the things that estrogen is good for.

You will have a nice, stable amount of hormones floating around — a greatly stabilizing factor on any of the symptoms that are caused by fluctuating levels of unopposed estrogen. In addition, the pills will eliminate menstrual concerns such as erratic periods or heavy bleeding. Your period will be very light and occur at a predictable time of the month, which is a big relief for many women.

The effect is physical and emotional. Some patients feel transformed:

*After taking Zoloft [an antidepressant] for a year for premenstrual mood swings and depression, I started taking Loestrin. It has been like a miracle. I went off it for a while, and the irritability started up right away.*

*At forty-nine, I experienced what were probably mild hot flashes. My FSH was on the border. My periods came and went with no rhyme or reason, but I still had them. I lost interest in everything — playing piano, my decorating, my work, my social life. I tried Loestrin first, but I felt dizzy. I tried Ortho-Cyclen. No more dizziness. I was amazed by the change in my mood. It was like someone turned on the lights.*

*I've lost nine pounds over the past three months with no change in eating or exercise habits. They say these pills don't do anything to your metabolism, but maybe when you feel better, when you have your energy back, it's just easier to stay on course.*

*We didn't want more children. I wanted a birth-control method I could count on. I'd had a horrible experience on birth-control pills in my twenties. I was bloated, depressed. I couldn't stay on them for a month. These low-dose pills were different. My moods no longer jumped all over the map. That sullen five-day bitchiness before my period disappeared. My energy level improved. I feel steady all month long. It's taken so much stress out of my life. I wish I had known.*

*I skipped a period. I figured no big deal. Then I had the period from hell. I thought I was hemorrhaging. Huge clots, running to the bathroom every hour. I never, ever wanted to go through something like that again. Since taking low-dose pills, I feel great. I'm sleeping better, I have more energy, and I feel allover better than I have for a couple of years. When I first started, I had bad headaches, and some breakthrough bleeding. That stopped after a couple of months.*

*During the past year and a half, I figured those ugly feelings and emotions were about my marriage, which was ending; my divorce, which made me feel I'd failed; the death of my father, totally unexpected. But aren't so many women dealing with this? Low-dose pills brought a normalcy to my life I haven't experienced for a long time. I can't attribute it to anything else, because life is still difficult.*

*There are no words to describe my years before menopause. The depression was the killer. They had me on Prozac.*

*I was living in the Midwest then. I went to a gynecologist in Chicago. She said, "You have a cyst on your ovary." There was ovarian cancer in my family. I wanted to have it out. I signed a paper saying she could give me a full hysterectomy. If there was anything unhealthy, I felt like, "Just get rid of it."*

*So out went the cyst, an ovary, and a tube. I went home the same day, with Tylenol and codeine, after such major surgery. I was in agony. My doctor told me later she was saving me money!*

*All of this and I didn't feel better. I went back to the gynecologist. My husband went with me. The doctor said in so many words that there was no such thing as premenopause or perimenopause, that it was all ridiculous. She was fifty-two and had been through the change herself. She said I should look at my stress level. Meanwhile, I was so depressed. I just lay in bed. I went back on Prozac, which I had taken after a miscarriage. That whole five years in Chicago is a blur.*

*I was forty-nine and back in New York when I first started taking Loestrin, and you can believe me when I say that pregnancy was the last thing on my mind. Within three days [of my being] on Loestrin, my boss said, "What happened? What did you do?" The change was amazing.*

*I'll say this to other women who might experience the same: I didn't see a way out. There was no one to say to me that it's okay, it's perimenopause. See a gynecologist who understands perimenopause. Don't waste time with anyone who tells you this is all in your head.*

*I worked out. I drank teas. I took vitamins. Low-dose birth-control pills gave me back my personality and my life. I can function. I work effectively again. My mind doesn't wander all over the place. My joints don't ache all the time. I'm only forty-three years old. I thought something was seriously wrong with me. Now people aren't afraid to approach me because I'll cry or explode at them. Herbs, vitamins, teas, and working out were not working for me.*

Will you have the same kind of results with low-dose birth-control pills? I know one thing for sure. If you are willing to go for a two-month trial and then reevaluate how you are feeling, you will know that whatever fatigue or depression or anxiety you are still feeling is not related to fluctuating levels of unopposed estrogen.

When you try low-dose birth-control pills for perimenopausal symptoms, three things can happen: You may feel great and be thrilled that you tried them. Or you may feel worse and stop. Or you may feel exactly the same. And if you feel exactly the same, you aren't going to continue, because why would you take a medication if you didn't feel any different?

You aren't going to feel better after just one pill or even one cycle. It's not the Pill that makes you feel better. It's what it does to your system's hormonal production.

## Why the Pill Works on Subtle Symptoms

You may wonder how women can take a pill that shuts off their ovulatory cycles and suppresses their hormone production and end up with better moods, more energy, more optimistic outlooks. Much is still being researched, and there is much we still don't know. By the time you reach menopause, medical science may have more information about the years before it. The study of perimenopause is still in its infancy. But there is news about low-dose birth-control pills and their effects that you may want to consider right now, regardless of your symptoms. These pills not only protect you against conception, but against cancer.

## Types of Birth-Control Pills

There are three basic types of birth-control pills available. They are:

- Monophasic. Loestrin, which I prescribe frequently, is one example of a monophasic pill. Every medicated pill you take for twenty-one days contains the same amount of estrogen and progesterone. Lo/Ovral, Ortho-Novum, Demulen, Alesse, and Ortho-Cyclen are other examples.
- Triphasic. Triphasil, Ortho-Novum 7/7/7, Ortho-Tri-Cyclen, Tri-Norinyl. These pills have the same amount of estrogen but vary the amount of progestogen delivered during the course of the month. These are not conducive to time switching (taking them for more than three weeks on and then one week off when you want to delay your period).
- Minipills. These pills only contain progestogen. You don't have as high a level of assurance that you won't get pregnant, and they do not control estrogen levels the way traditional pills do. However, they are prescribed sometimes for birth control in women who can't take estrogen.

I prefer the monophasics because you get the *same* dose of estrogen and progesterone for the entire package.

## Birth-Control Pills Can Provide Cancer Prevention

It is a sad fact that most women in the United States are not aware that oral contraceptives provide protection against ovarian and endometrial cancer.

Studies indicate that only one year of oral contraceptive use reduces the risk of endometrial cancer (uterine cancer) by 50 percent. This protection lasts for at least fifteen years after discontinuation of the medication!

After five years of use, the risk of ovarian cancer is diminished by 50 percent. Significant protection against ovarian cancer is gained with as little as six months of use. The longer the use, the greater the protection.

Although the incidence of ovarian cancer is only half that of endometrial cancer, it is the fourth leading cause of cancer mortality in women in the United States. This is due to the difficulty of early diagnosis and the lack of effective treatment.

In the Centers for Disease Control and Prevention's multifaceted Cancer and Steroid Hormone (CASH) study, the largest such study to date, the risk of endometrial cancer was reduced overall by 40 percent in women taking low-dose birth-control pills. The same study found that ovarian cancer risk began to drop as early as three to six months after the Pill was started.

## Benefits of Ultra-Low-Dose Birth-Control Pills Go Far Beyond Their Ability to Prevent a Late Pregnancy

Other benefits of low-dose birth-control pills for older women include the following:

- Less benign breast disease. Women taking birth-control pills have a 35 to 50 percent decrease in fibrocystic breast disease.
- Fewer ovarian cysts. Researchers estimate that women using oral contraceptives are 70 percent less likely to develop benign ovarian cysts.
- Fewer ectopic pregnancies. Ectopic pregnancies occur when the fertilized egg remains in the fallopian tube instead of moving into

the uterus. Eventually the pregnancy can burst the tube, ending the pregnancy and also causing severe abdominal pain and quite often serious internal hemorrhaging.

- More regular menses. Pill users enjoy less flow and fewer PMS symptoms.
- Less iron-deficiency anemia. Because the Pill causes less flow during your period, it is estimated that women who use it are half as likely to develop iron-deficiency anemia as women who don't take the Pill.
- Less pelvic inflammatory disease. PID is a bacterial infection that occurs when bacteria enter the uterus and spread to the fallopian tubes, ovaries, and surrounding tissue. Generally, the bacteria are introduced during sexual intercourse. PID can cause severe pain in the lower abdomen as well as heavy, irregular bleeding. Birth-control pill users have a lower risk of contracting PID, perhaps because the Pill thickens cervical mucus, which may provide protection against bacteria.
- Less rheumatoid arthritis
- Increased bone density. Bone density peaks by age thirty-five to forty. The higher the peak, the better off you'll be at age sixty, seventy, and eighty.

## What You Need to Know Before You Go on the Pill

The list of side effects of the Pill, which arise most often during the first few months of use, has remained virtually unchanged in recent years. The package insert will warn you of headache, nausea and vomiting, acne, weight gain, breast tenderness and enlargement, vision changes, depression, and spotting. But with the lower doses, acne and weight gain are much less likely than with the older versions of the Pill. In fact, the progestin in Ortho-Cyclen (relatively new) is now labeled by the FDA as a treatment for acne!

The side effects that alarm my patients most are very scanty periods and breakthrough bleeding. After heavy periods that sent you running to the bathroom every hour, these scant periods can seem unusual. But they are normal. The uterine lining doesn't build up much on the Pill.

If you miss a pill, the balance of hormones is so delicate that you may well experience breakthrough bleeding. You may experience it anyway. Breakthrough bleeding is annoying, but it doesn't mean that your health is at risk. A higher dose pill — not too much higher and nothing near the birth-control pills you took in your twenties — can counter breakthrough bleeding. Some patients would rather stick with the lower dose and deal with the bleeding. Others are ready to go up one level to see if it helps.

Who should not take the Pill? Smokers who are over thirty-five years old. Women with a history of phlebitis or pulmonary emboli (blood clots in the lungs). If you are taking anticonvulsants, inform your doctor, because there may be a drug interaction with the Pill.

People with high blood pressure are not usually prescribed the Pill. However, in order to be properly diagnosed with hypertension, women should have their blood pressure checked on multiple occasions. They need to make sure when these tests are given that they are not taking any medications, including over-the-counter medications. In my experience, many over-the-counter medications, especially cold remedies, can result in transient changes in blood pressure. Before I will label a patient as having hypertension and suggest treatment for it, I feel her pressure should be checked on at least three occasions. I recommend that patients have readings done on days when they feel particularly relaxed and haven't had a cup of coffee that morning. If two of those three measurements are elevated, I am comfortable diagnosing hypertension and would agree that this is a reason not to be on birth-control pills.

Women with fibroids often ask if they should not be taking the Pill. Fibroids clearly respond to estrogen. They do not appear prior to menarche, the first period, and after natural menopause, fibroids almost invariably decrease in size. However, the amount of estrogen and progesterone in birth-control pills is often quite a bit lower than the amount that women who are anovulatory make naturally.

I discuss fibroids in detail in chapter 7. I explain why women who have the type of fibroids known as "intramural" and "subserosal" fibroids along with dysfunctional anovulatory bleeding actually benefit tremendously from cycle regulation with low-dose birth-control pills. In any case, most of the time fibroids do not grow from low-dose birth-control pills and are not a contraindication for women who want to try them.

## Breast Cancer and the Pill

Your doctor recommends low-dose birth-control pills, but you're reluctant to try them. Fear of breast cancer may be your number one worry. The 17.5 million American women taking the Pill are anxious for answers about the possible relationship between birth-control pills and breast cancer. There have been numerous studies conducted around the world. In the early nineties, studies contradicted other studies. Every study was a media event, and bad news about the side effects of birth-control pills tended to travel faster than good.

A study in June of 1995 published in the *New England Journal of Medicine* followed 122,000 nurses for fourteen years. The conclusion was that hormone replacement therapy (not equivalent to birth-control pills!) increased the risk of breast cancer by 30 to 40 percent.

Then came a study in July of the same year in the *Journal of the American Medical Association.* This study compared 500 women aged fifty to sixty-four who had been diagnosed with breast cancer to a control group of healthy women. That study found no link between the use of hormone replacement therapy and breast cancer. The researchers even found that women who had used hormones for eight years or longer had a lower risk of breast cancer than those who had never taken them.

The fact that two such large studies contradicted each other only confused people, and researchers still argue about the interpretations of both studies. Again, these studies were looking at hormone replacement therapy, *not* low-dose birth-control pills — not a subtle difference but a material one. (I discuss the risks versus the benefits of hormone replacement therapy in chapter 11.)

If there were a large risk of breast cancer among women who use hormonal contraceptives or hormone replacement therapy, you have to wonder why such a risk would not have been identified more easily. Still, a weak link isn't no link when you're a woman considering low-dose birth-control pills. Women tend to link hormone replacement therapy drugs with birth-control pills when they are two very different things. A woman taking birth-control pills, for example, usually has less estrogen in her body than if she allowed nature to take its course. She is not adding estrogen to her body, but turning off her natural supply and adding a measured, healthy amount.

The most recent and best data indicate that there is no increased risk of breast cancer from birth-control pill use. Research published in the journal *Contraception* in 1996 has gone far toward providing a clear-cut answer. Two hundred researchers brought together virtually all the studies ever done on the subject. The research included 153,536 women from twenty-five countries who had been on the Pill.

Their conclusion? There is no increased chance of being diagnosed with breast cancer ten to twenty years after stopping the use of the Pill. This was true whether or not women had a family history of breast cancer. It held regardless of ethnic group, whether or not a woman had natural children, the number of years a woman used the Pill, or the type of dosage.

An interesting finding was that women in the study who used the Pill and did develop breast cancer were more likely than nonusers to have localized tumors that had not spread beyond the breast and were more easily treated. This may be because women on the Pill are more likely to be seeing a doctor on a regular basis and have better surveillance, catching breast tumors earlier.

## What to Do if You Choose to Take the Pill

Doctors ensure maximum safety for their patients taking birth-control pills by monitoring them regularly. Here's what you can do to maximize your success and lessen any risks:

1) Don't ignore your regular checkups. I recommend that all women in transition see their gynecologists two times a year instead of annually, and I feel this is especially important for women on the Pill.

2) Ask for the lowest-dose pill and see if that solves the problem. Loestrin 1/20 has 20 mcg of ethinyl estradiol. Alesse, a newer brand on the market, has the same 20 mcg of ethinyl estradiol, but a different progestin (levonorgesterol). Ortho-Cyclen differs slightly from

both. It has more estrogen, 35 mcg, but uses a newer progesterone, norgestimate, that seems to have fewer side effects. The differences in ingredients are subtle, but the effects can be monumental in that you can feel bloated and uncomfortable on one pill and find that another completely relieves those symptoms.

You might have to undergo some fine-tuning of your medication to get the best results. For example, there are patients who do well the three weeks they are taking the medication but complain of symptoms in the week off the pills. I and other doctors have begun to allow such patients to take up to six weeks of medication and then one week of withdrawal in order to minimize their suffering. This may sound strange at first, but think back to when you were younger and taking the Pill, and you wanted to avoid having your period on your honeymoon or an important vacation. Your doctor may have told you to keep taking the Pill for an extra week to forestall your period. There's no danger in doing this. One of the wonderful things about the Pill is that because the period you get is artificial, you can shift it when you need to.

3) Get regular mammograms — something every woman in transition should do anyway. Don't forget to do your own monthly self-exams the week after your period begins.

4) If you have heavy bleeding between periods, phone your doctor. This is not the same as spotting. Midcycle spotting is common when women first take the Pill. Fifteen to twenty percent of women have it when they first begin taking low-dose pills. Sometimes the estrogen in the Pill cannot maintain the lining of the endometrium at first. It becomes destabilized, and you spot. Another brand of pill may be worth a try. In any case, your body may take several months to adjust. After two months of midcycle spotting you should reevaluate your experience with your doctor.

## What You Can Do if You Can't (Or Don't Want to) Take the Pill

Many women can recall a time in their youth when they didn't get their period for months, went to the doctor, and were given some pills that brought on their period. These pills were usually some type of synthetic progesterone. To understand what progesterone does, recall that estrogen makes the lining (endometrium) of the uterus thick. After ovulation the follicle converts to the corpus luteum. It secretes progesterone, which encourages the growth of blood vessels and glands so that the uterus is prepared to receive a fertilized egg. If fertilization does not occur, this lining will be shed. In perimenopause, however, if a woman doesn't ovulate, there is no progesterone to do this job. This can result in abnormal bleeding patterns.

Without progesterone, the endometrium will keep growing. When it's finally destabilized and shed, you can have a very heavy bleed. Also, progesterone is known to help prevent endometrial cancer. An endometrium that is growing unchecked can lead to hyperplasia, a breeding ground for precancerous changes.

Progestins can be prescribed to regulate the cycle and protect you. Progesterone is a natural substance made by your ovaries, while progestogen and progestins are synthetic substances that have a progesterone-like effect. Women who cannot or are very reluctant to take oral contraceptive pills can be cycled with medroxyprogesterone acetate, a progestin that goes by the brand name Provera, as well as Cycrin. Provera is the most widely used progestin in the U.S.A., with a long track record of safety. (Provera is also often given to women after menopause as part of hormone replacement therapy, which I discuss in chapter 11.) Patients take 5 to 10 mg per day for ten to fourteen days per month.

Although Provera will regulate your bleeding, it may not have as great an effect as low-dose birth-control pills on the psychosocial symptoms that occur in perimenopause. Sometimes it makes symptoms like breast tenderness and bloating worse because it can cause water retention. Sometimes women complain of nausea. Many women complain of mood swings. If this should occur, see if trying another brand of progestin helps. Lowering the dose can also minimize side effects.

## What's Ahead: Crinone, an Exciting New Alternative

Crinone has recently become available in the United States. It is a form of natural progesterone that can be delivered in a gel placed in the vagina. It comes in single-dose applicators used at bedtime ten nights per month. It is a great alternative for patients who don't want to take oral progestin.

Unlike vaginal creams for treating infections, which involve a large applicator and are often quite messy, this gel comes in an applicator the size of a thimble. The major advantage of this form of progesterone is that it is absorbed well into the uterus and thus protects against the unopposed estrogen effects of hyperplasia and cancers. Because there isn't significant systemic absorption (meaning through the liver and then through all of your tissues), it does not result in any of the other symptoms often attributed to Provera (breast tenderness, mood swings, bloating). The use of this vaginal progesterone gel should result in elimination of most abnormal dysfunctional uterine bleeding.

Crinone, like all progesterone agents, is an option for smokers, as well as women with high blood pressure.

## Questions Women Ask

*I never had PMS until I was thirty-eight. Now, two days before my period, it gets to the point where I feel almost suicidal. I feel better the moment I start to bleed. I've thought about going on low-dose birth-control pills just to get me through two days of every month when I'm basically fine otherwise. Is it worth it?*

The obvious question is Why not? Do you want to get pregnant? If you don't, there is absolutely no overall health advantage for spitting out an egg every twenty-eight days. There is nothing inherently advantageous about bursting the capsule of your ovary and having to repair it each month. There's no reason for having fluctuating levels of hormones floating around unless you want to have a baby. This may seem hard to believe, but it's true.

I am amazed at how often somebody who has the same doubts you have calls up at the end of two months on low-dose birth-control pills and says, "I can't believe how great I feel. I can't believe I didn't do this five years ago. I thought I just had crummy PMS. I feel much more stable all month long. And my periods are really light. This is great."

There is nothing wrong with choosing to ride out the storm without medication But low-dose cycle regulators offer many women much-sought-after relief.

> *When I'm on low-dose birth-control pills is there anything I should be doing to counteract any side effects?*

Stay away from salt. Breast tenderness, headaches, and bloated feelings are the result of water retention in different organ systems. Water retention in the breast results in breast tenderness. Water retention in the gut results in a bloated feeling. When patients complain to me about side effects of the Pill, many of them are due to salt.

I also recommend using time-release vitamin $B_6$. Many women report that it markedly diminishes side effects. Choose the time-release 200-mg dose. Otherwise you will urinate it away in four hours.

> *I have a problem with taking medication for something that isn't a disease. How do we know that women aren't supposed to have perimenopause for some positive reason? By taking pills, aren't we messing around with nature?*

More likely, nature is messing around with you! The debate about whether women should intervene in the reproductive cycle at all has been going on since most of us were in our teens, when the first birth-control pill was invented. Many of my patients are reluctant to undergo cycle regulation. Their feeling is "I would like to leave it to nature." You should be aware of the following facts:

We live in a society that is far removed from "nature." Because we are living so long and have access to many kinds of birth control, a woman today may have hundreds more menstrual cycles in her lifetime than her ancestors did. Consider, for argument's sake, a woman who begins her period at age ten and ends at age fifty. She would have forty years, each of which has thirteen lunar months, of cycles: 520 in all.

Two thousand years ago, which is a drop in the bucket in terms of evolution, a woman might have had eight children. That is nine cycles eliminated per child — seventy-two total. She would have nursed those kids for up to fifteen months each (no formula, no bottles, etc.), and that deletes another 120 cycles. In all probability, she would have had three pregnancy losses, accounting for another six cycles apiece (totaling eighteen). The total number of cycles that would be eliminated over her lifetime is approximately 210. Many women today will have two children and either not nurse or nurse for three or four months, eliminating 24 cycles instead of 210. My point is that it is not "natural" to have 520 cycles in one's lifetime — it's a phenomenon of the last few decades.

I have long believed that these extra ovulatory cycles have a link to increased risk of ovarian cancer. Recall that when you ovulate, you burst the ovarian capsule to discharge an egg. Eighty-five percent of ovarian tumors are of the epithelium, which is the capsule layer that covers the ovary. This is the part that bursts and repairs, bursts and repairs with ovulation. Many tumors in the body occur at areas of active growth and repair (for instance, the cervix, at the junction where new tissue is constantly being laid down). This may be why women who take birth-control pills, which inhibit ovulation and thus the burst and repair of the capsules, have a decreased incidence of ovarian cancer.

New studies are beginning to provide proof of this theory. In a 1997 study, Joellen M. Schildkraut, Ph.D., and colleagues at the Duke University Medical Center concluded that the more times a woman ovulates over her lifetime, the greater the chance that a key gene called p53, which is thought to suppress tumor growth, will mutate, be transformed, and permit the formation of ovarian cancer. These mutations occur because in order for the ruptured ovarian surface to repair itself after ovulation, cellular proliferation that can cause DNA damage is required.

One can look upon pregnancy and nursing as "nature's" method of cycle suppression. Since you don't enter pregnancy or lactation as often or for as long as "nature" intended you to, it may make the best medical sense to put yourself into a state of cycle suppression with birth-control pills, or "cycle regulators."

I admit that I am not a believer in letting nature take its course, whether it has to do solely with a woman's menstrual cycle, or with her overall health and well-being. The longer my patients live, the less medical sense I see in letting nature have the last word if it means pain or poor health. My job as a doctor is to help prevent and remove suffering. For every woman, the issue is choice.

*I'm feeling so good on low-dose pills. But I'm going to be fifty-one next week. I'm reluctant to switch and try something that won't work as well as the pills I've been on. How long can one stay on these pills?*

When a patient is doing well with cycle regulation on a pill that contains 20 mcg of estrogen, I anticipate her staying on it right into menopause. When she reaches somewhere around age fifty, I start to check FSH levels on the sixth day of the pill-free week. If FSH levels are elevated, I may recommend that the patient transfer to traditional hormone replacement therapy. However, many of my patients are fifty and doing so well on their low-dose pills that they can continue slightly longer before switching. I am reluctant to change much of anything simply because a woman has hit some magical number of fifty years of age.

*I am going to quit smoking. How long until I can take the Pill?*

You don't want to begin the Pill while you're still at a delicate point in your smoking cessation program. The danger is relapse. It sometimes goes like this: You have one or two cigarettes when you're out with friends. The next day you quit again. Then you find you're smoking a couple a day. Somehow that turns into half a pack. You don't want to be a smoker on low-dose birth-control pills. Once you're confident that your chances of relapse are remote, you can be an excellent candidate for low-dose pills.

*Will I ever know if I go into menopause if I'm taking birth-control pills?*

There are tests that can tell you if you are menopausal, and you can request them. If they show that you're in menopause, you should be switched to the more physiologically appropriate hormone replacement therapy. Premarin is the most common estrogen prescribed. There are also new drugs coming out on the market called SERMs, which I discuss in chapter 11. Your youth is on your side in terms of hormone replacement therapy options.

*I've read that by taking low-dose birth-control pills, you can skip menopause altogether. Is that true?*

Can you skip the eventual end of ovulation and your ability to reproduce? No. But many women confuse menopause with perimenopause. They think of the symptoms, the hormonal ups and downs, as menopause. *The transition to menopause is often worse than menopause.* Clinically, menopause means that menstruation has stopped for at least six months, given, of course, that you're at the appropriate age. At that point, you're usually done with subtle symptoms and menstrual problems. Hot flashes and dry vagina signal that actual menopause is very close, because these symptoms are related to the fact that your body is no longer making estrogen. Low-dose birth-control pills ameliorate these symptoms by taking control of ovaries that are functioning erratically and providing steady doses of hormones. At the time of actual menopause, you will need to make the decision about hormone replacement therapy (HRT).

> *I never used birth-control pills before. It seems strange to use them now, especially since my husband has had a vasectomy.*

Think of them as "cycle regulators," not birth-control pills. How bad are your symptoms? Many patients are using them for the first time in their late thirties and early forties because of enhanced premenstrual syndrome. Or they have had light periods for years and now are having very heavy ones. Or they are developing anovulatory bleeding.

Ten years ago what we had to offer these patients was a D&C (dilation and curettage) or a hysterectomy. It is much safer to be taking low-dose birth-control pills.

> *I went on low-dose pills because of terrible mood swings. They are somewhat improved, but I still have them. Should I take a stronger pill?*

If a patient is finding her swings are somewhat improved on a low-dose pill, I often will try her on an alternative low-dose pill, either with a different progesterone or perhaps a slightly different dose of estrogen. Often the best pill for a particular patient is determined by trial and error. Realize that it is unlikely that any medication is going to result in 100 percent improvement. I often explain to patients that whatever symptoms they are having may be a complex interaction between hormonal balance (or lack thereof) and life events. I feel confident that whatever component of their psychosocial symptoms are hormonally mediated can be eliminated through cycle regulation with low-dose birth-control pills.

*What if I choose to do nothing about perimenopause?*
You can. The first option I offer a woman who is experiencing perimenopausal symptoms is that she can do nothing. She can take this
new understanding about her body and how it works and see if that is
enough to dispel the anxiety. My experience has made me aware of
how strong the mind-body connection really is. Once you know why
you're feeling tired or cranky, or what that funny bleeding is about,
you may be able to cope without medication. Probably 60 percent of
my patients who learn they are in perimenopause go forward without
medication. For them, simply understanding *why* they feel the way
they do gives them a reassurance that is itself a very powerful "medicine." Furthermore, I make them understand that if they want to go
further, medications are available. This doesn't make them good patients or bad patients. There's no judgment here. Every woman must
consider what's right for her.

Knowing what is going on in your body and choosing to do nothing isn't the same as suffering in silence not knowing why you feel the
way you do.

*I'm not closed to the idea of estrogen replacement therapy when I
really need it after menopause. But I don't want to take any
medication now. What are the most important alternatives you
would suggest for women like me?*
Here are some ways you can try to control symptoms and stay healthy
if you don't want to use birth-control pills, progestin, or any other
medication.

1) If you smoke, you must find a way to stop.
2) Exercise regularly.
3) Reduce your stress through relaxation. Massage, hot baths, and
meditation can all be helpful on a regular basis.
4) Modify your diet to reduce fat. Eat plenty of carbohydrates.
Some researchers suggest that eating carbohydrates boosts serotonin
levels, which can help steady mood swings. Don't indulge in too
much liquor, coffee, chocolate, soda, or salt. Caffeine increases the
loss of calcium. Chocolate and other high-fat items contribute to

weight gain and heart disease. Salt raises blood pressure, not to mention its water-retentive powers.

5) Take vitamins; 400 IU vitamin D, 1,000–2,000 mg time-release vitamin C, 10,000 IU vitamin A, and 200 mg time-release $B_6$. Patients sometimes ask me if it's better to get these vitamins through food than vitamin pills. It's great if you can get everything you need from food, but it's difficult to quantify, and most people fall far short. If the vitamins you take are water soluble, any excess will be urinated away and will not cause you any problem.

6) Increase calcium. Don't wait until menopause.

7) Go to the doctor for routine checkups.

8) Do monthly breast exams.

9) Ask your parents or other relatives about anything in the family medical history that might be pertinent. You'd be surprised at how many women have no clue because they don't want to "talk about these things." Knowledge is power.

10) Don't take every symptom you have as something you must deal with on your own because you don't want to be a complainer. Maybe you pride yourself on the fact that you can handle things well with a couple of aspirin, but consider this: Subtle symptoms often help a doctor discover a bigger picture. Don't automatically conclude that "This is no big deal." Make the most of every annual visit.

11) Take control of your medical appointment. I discuss how you can get the best out of an annual exam at great length in chapter 8, but the summary is this: You have to take increasing control of your health care in the era of managed care. You will get the most out of every medical appointment by seeing yourself and your doctor as a team. You need to be prepared rather than passive. That takes knowledge on your part. It takes the kind of assertiveness that you build by becoming knowledgeable about your body and how it works.

# 4

# SHOULD YOU TREAT YOUR SYMPTOMS NATURALLY?

Patients often tell me they are very concerned about the side effects of drugs. They want to know about a more "natural" approach to health. But does natural really mean better?

Botanical remedies, relatively new to the U.S.A., are usually what patients mean when they talk about natural remedies. These botanicals have wider acceptance in Europe and many other countries than they do here. As they become more in vogue across the world, I want my patients to be as educated about them as I would want them to be about taking Ortho-Cyclen or another low-dose pill. You need to consider all the information and decide which approach or combination of approaches meets your needs best.

## A Warning About "Natural" Remedies for Perimenopause

The first "natural remedies" you are going to encounter when you begin to become conscious of perimenopause and do some reading are usually dong quai, black cohosh, primrose oil, and yam roots. You'll also hear a lot about soy.

The most important point to remember is this: Perimenopause isn't menopause. Unfortunately, the terms perimenopause, pre-menopause, menopause, and postmenopause often get thrown around as if they were all the same. Doctors confuse them, so there's no reason the media, your friends, and family wouldn't use them interchangeably. The thinking goes: Such and such helps women in menopause, so it's bound to be even better in perimenopause, at the start. It's all the same thing, right?

Wrong. Perimenopause is a very distinct stage in a woman's body that requires health strategies geared to what's going on hormonally at that time. Your best friend, ten years older than you, may be helped by remedies she buys over the counter at the health-food store that would make your symptoms worse. She may have stopped menstruating two years ago. Her body has stopped making estrogen.

More simply, what your body needs to relieve the symptoms of perimenopause is quite different from what you need once your body stops making estrogen. One patient's story is a case in point. I don't think Sharon, forty-five, had slept through the night for three weeks when I first saw her. The circles under her eyes were deep purple. When she walked into my consultation room prior to her exam and shook my hand, I noticed polished nails, but her cuticles looked ragged and bloody.

Still, she had a manner that spoke of quiet strength in spite of bone-tired weariness. It had taken courage to consult a doctor. It had taken her two years.

Two years ago, her aunt's bout with terminal bladder cancer made her abandon what had once been a pretty consistent schedule of annual gynecological visits. "My aunt's case was badly handled," she says. "Even the last doctor we consulted told us so. But it was too late. I was very close to her. Maybe there was nothing they could really do, but it seemed that everything she endured in the hospital made it worse. She was a vital, active, wonderful woman before her cancer was diagnosed. It was downhill from the moment she started treatment.

"The whole family turned against doctors. We didn't talk to other people who were going through the same thing. It isn't my family's way. We talked to each other. We just got more angry, more desperate. I mean, you grasp at straws.

"In the middle of all of this, I started not getting my period. Last month I had a massive period. The cramps lasted two weeks and they were so bad I had to stay in bed. I was changing a tampon every hour. Now I'm having cramps again. I'm having everything I usually have, but my period hasn't come."

I asked if she was taking any medications. "No medicine. But my cousin told me about black cohosh. It's something you get at health-food stores. She started seeing an herbalist for her arthritis. She swears by him. He told her about black cohosh when she started having hot flashes, and ever since she's been feeling great. He said it could regulate a woman's cycle. Anyway, that's what I've been taking for the last year."

I asked if she was having trouble sleeping. "I wake up at three in the morning, and I can't go back. Finally, I fall asleep around six A.M. and can't wake up at seven. I tried melatonin, and it was okay. But then I have weeks where nothing works. I'm just so jumpy all the time."

One of the things that was keeping her awake was worry over the heavy bleeding followed by no bleeding. "Do you think it could be cancer?" she asked me.

Sharon was feeling horrible, and there were excellent medical reasons why. Here was a woman whose tests showed she was clearly perimenopausal. For her cousin, who was ten years older and in menopause, black cohosh made some sense, since it contains phytoesterols, which have estrogen-like effects. Sharon's medical problems were different. Her body was still making estrogen. But she wasn't ovulating regularly, so she wasn't making any progesterone. Black cohosh was giving her the opposite of what her body needed. The sleeplessness became more pronounced as her body tried to cope with even more estrogen without progesterone to balance it.

Sharon's case is one extreme, but it can happen to any woman. In the health-food stores I've visited, these drugs are often grouped in the "women's health" section. There is nothing to indicate what is helpful before menopause or after it, as if every "female problem" is the same thing.

## Natural or Risk Free?

There is no question that there are herbs and extracts that are potent. They're called phytoestrogens. These are "plant estrogens," which appear to have plant hormones or hormone precursors in them.

But just because they come from plants and are available at health-food stores is no reason to think any of them is preferable to medication that is FDA regulated, tested on thousands of women, and successful with millions of patients. *Just because it comes from nature doesn't make it better.* As a doctor, I spend a lot of time trying to circumvent nature. Nature can be very cruel. Nature lets mothers die in childbirth.

Women sometimes ask me about natural remedies when it isn't really natural they're interested in but risk free. If you think you are going to avoid the risk of breast cancer — or any other side effect, real or media hyped — by using these "natural" remedies, this is the reality: If it's stopping your hot flashes, if it's affecting your body, it's affecting your breasts.

If you're in menopause and you've come to the conclusion that you are going to take estrogen, you should know what dose you're taking. If you are in perimenopause, and your symptoms are caused by unopposed estrogen, you could put yourself at risk by adding even more estrogen to your body.

I'm a man of medicine, but I can understand that people have become disillusioned with modern drugs because of their high cost, inability to cure everything, and side effects. But botanicals don't offer miracle answers, either. Most of what you will find at the health-food store in the "midlife woman's section" are nothing more than diluted medications that happen to come from plants. I worry about women bypassing the safeguards of modern medicine and diagnosing and medicating themselves.

The issue isn't just that these remedies aren't backed by enough scientific evidence to show that they work. These botanicals are not subject to the same intense scrutiny the FDA mandates for prescription drugs, because although they are touted as drugs, they aren't labeled as such. Manufacturers are not required to test products for safety and purity. Herbal laxative teas, for example, are widely available in health-food stores. At least four women have died and many have become ill from drinking them. I want to be assured of some quality control in any substance that passes through my liver, and you should too. There's little out there that insures the quality of these over-the-counter herbs. Equally important, botanicals do not have magical powers. You cannot "kick" your body into producing hormones you lack by taking passion flower or whatever.

The botanicals that are most widely touted for menopausal symptoms are the ones that contain plant estrogens, or phytoestrogens. Herbalists claim that phytoestrogens can raise a woman's low level of estrogen and also lower a high level by replacing a stronger form of estrogen with a weaker one. They don't turn off your natural production of hormones, however.

For many of my perimenopausal patients, estrogen is not the only problem. This is a time of hormonal unbalance, with another culprit being a lack of progesterone to offset the estrogen. The last thing you need to do at this point is add additional estrogen in any form.

If you are intent on trying botanicals, educate yourself — and don't depend on the person behind the counter to inform you. He or she may have been hired last week and given no training at all, unlike your pharmacist, who has undergone years of specialized training.

## Botanicals, Oils, and Veggie Remedies: Will They Work for You?

The following are the most commonly recommended panaceas for gynecological problems and my thoughts about each.

### Dong Quai (Angelica Sinesis)

Also known as Chinese angelica root, this is one of the most widely used herbs in Chinese traditional medicine and contains phytoestrogens. It is purported to relieve hot flashes, vaginal dryness, and depression. It supposedly works by promoting the body's use of and response to available estrogen. It can be taken as a liquid that can be added to water. About thirty drops daily is the usual dosage. Or it can be taken as thin slices of cured root. "It increases the effectiveness of the estrogen that now is released primarily from a woman's fat tissue after menopause," one herbalist told me. Depending on whom you talk to, dong quai can cure all "female complaints," from looking pale to having cramps. I have a problem with that, given the lack of studies proving it to be effective at doing anything.

THE BOTTOM LINE: You're taking estrogen. It will be metabolized in your liver and function in your body very similarly to estrogens that are synthetic. If you're in perimenopause and still making estrogen, you don't need more.

I've heard this scenario more than once: "I've been taking this thing [dong quai, herbs, green tea, whatever], and it worked at first. Then it didn't work, so I started taking more. In a couple of months it started working again."

Maybe so, but if you are perimenopausal and had that experience, it was probably because you finally had an ovulatory cycle. Your symptoms disappeared. You thought, "Finally, this dong quai is starting to work." More likely, your ovary released an egg. Progesterone combated all that estrogen in your body and gave you a sense of balance again.

Perimenopausal patients who take dong quai hoping it will combat their heavy bleeding often find that it makes their bleeding worse. They're adding this there and that here when the balance is already precarious. Remember that hormonal imbalance isn't the symptom but the cause. That's why birth-control pills work so well. They shut off your unbalanced hormone production and give you steady amounts of estrogen and progesterone all month long. I have serious doubts that you can get that kind of balance from dong quai. There is a great variability in the potency among different samples of the herb. Even for my menopausal patients who need to add estrogen to their systems, my biggest problem is what dose are they getting?

THE GRAIN OF TRUTH: Natural can be potent. Many active substances have been isolated from dong quai. Some are antiseptic, anti-allergic, stimulant, analgesic, anti-inflammatory. There is plenty of anecdotal evidence that dong quai helps hot flashes. Women having hot flashes are generally quite near actual menopause and may find that the estrogenic properties of dong quai help. When you are closer to actual menopause and no longer making estrogen, which you can find out from blood tests administered by your doctor, you might find dong quai useful. You may do better with herbs that are not estrogenic but still relieve your symptoms. In any case, dong quai is nontoxic and may boost energy because of its stimulant properties.

## Black Cohosh (Cimicifuga Racemosa, Also Squawroot)
Black cohosh is also known as black snakeroot. This is a plant, available as an extract, that is purported to supply estrogenic sterols —

the building blocks for estrogen, progesterone, and testosterone. It grew wild in the Ohio River Valley and was used by American Indian women there. I've heard naturalists say that when the pituitary is "screaming" for estrogen, black cohosh is perceived by the body as a breakdown product of estrogen. This supposedly signals the hypothalamus that there is enough estrogen in the system and to stop pumping out the FSH. It has also been suggested for the treatment of high blood pressure, anxiety, cramps, bronchitis, and fever.

THE BOTTOM LINE: I don't know about "screaming" pituitary glands, but I do know that research has shown estrogenic activity in women taking the herb. It appears to reduce the frequency of hot flashes in menopausal women.

Be that as it may, before you use black cohosh, a diagnosis of what's causing your problems is key. Are you truly menopausal and thus lacking estrogen? Or are you perimenopausal and dealing with fluctuating levels of unopposed estrogen as your cycle goes awry? You need a medical evaluation to determine this.

In any case, avoid black cohosh if you think there is any chance you might become pregnant or if you're trying to become pregnant. Avoid it if you are bleeding heavily; it can make your bleeding worse.

There are no studies of the herb's effect when it's taken for years at a time. Women starting black cohosh in their perimenopausal years and keeping at it into menopause may be taking a major risk.

THE GRAIN OF TRUTH: If this in fact functions as an estrogen, women who are menopausal and are no longer making estrogen may get a benefit. A study of eighty women in Germany found that those taking black cohosh reported the same reduction of symptoms as those taking Premarin, while the group taking a placebo reported the least change. However, doctors prescribe progesterone for twelve days each month along with estrogen for menopause to protect the uterus from hyperplasia. Women taking plant estrogens alone run a major risk from hyperplasia.

In any case, black cohosh isn't going to do anything for fluctuating levels of unopposed estrogen in women who are anovulatory, except add more estrogen. It's a mild diuretic, however, which may account for its popularity among women who struggle with bloating.

## Blue Cohosh (Caulophyllum Thalictroides)

Blue cohosh is recommended for the same ailments black cohosh is. It is often purported to be "more of the same" for women taking black cohosh, i.e., here's one more treatment for menstrual problems.

**THE BOTTOM LINE:** Danger. Blue cohosh contains caulosaponin. This is a substance that can raise blood pressure, cause digestive problems such as intestinal spasms, and constrict the blood vessels leading to the heart. "Natural" can be potent.

**THE GRAIN OF TRUTH:** I couldn't find one. My advice is don't take it — period.

## Ginseng (Panax Schinseng)

Said to help maintain energy and youthfulness, and even heighten sex drive, ginseng has been used in traditional Chinese herbal medicine for over five thousand years. Some say it helps them recover from illnesses such as the common cold and helps combat fatigue. Women have become especially interested in it lately because it is said to help control hot flashes and have estrogenic properties.

**THE BOTTOM LINE:** There are two types of ginseng: American and Chinese or Korean. There are also ginseng teas, candies, and dried roots. Many of these contain little if any ginseng at all.

I warn perimenopausal women against ginseng for several reasons. First of all, ginseng is a potent estrogen plant. Second, the Asian kind especially is a stimulant. If you are dealing with insomnia, irritability, or free-floating anxiety, this may exacerbate your problem. In some women it raises blood pressure. It is also not advised for women who might become pregnant.

**THE GRAIN OF TRUTH:** If you can get good ginseng from a reputable supplier, are in menopause, and are looking for a stimulant to boost your vitality, ginseng may sound like the very thing you've been looking for. However, you will have to take your chances on how much estrogen you are getting and take progesterone at the same time so that you don't run the risk of endometrial cancer.

## Wild Yam Root

Wild yam root is said to regulate the menstrual cycle. Sometimes it is irresponsibly suggested as a birth-control method.

THE BOTTOM LINE: No mystery here. All of the synthetic hormones except Premarin, including other estrogens, progesterone, progestin, and testosterone, are made from wild yam root. In fact, wild yam was once the sole source of chemicals used as raw materials in the manufacture of the Pill.

The extract from wild yam root is sometimes said to be a type of progesterone. Women who are menopausal and are prescribed progesterone because it protects the uterus from cancer sometimes have a problem with side effects. They may turn to yam extract in hopes that they'll have a better reaction to it. It's true that the extract contains diosgenin, used in making synthetic hormones, but there is no evidence that the human body can convert diosgenin to hormones.

If your doctor recommends that you take progesterone and you want to go the "natural" route, there are many other natural progesterones on the market that will be more effective than yam root for this purpose. They are made individually, not by national pharmaceutical firms.

THE GRAIN OF TRUTH: Yams, not the same as wild yam root, are rich sources of beta carotene and vitamins C and B$_6$. They are also high in fiber. There are benefits to including them in your diet for those reasons alone.

## Flaxseed Oil

Flaxseed oil is very rich in the omega-3 fatty acids thought to be important to heart health and blood pressure. Omega-3s are said to lower triglyceride levels as well as decrease the probability of a blood clot blocking an artery. In addition, omega-3s are said to decrease allergic responses.

Flaxseed is also a source of phytoestrogens, similar to soy. I have heard women say that their premenstrual syndromes and menopausal

symptoms are completely relieved within one month of flax inges-
tion, and that their vitality improves.

**THE BOTTOM LINE:** Here is another instance where I can't recommend the remedy without more scientific scrutiny. If you're using it
and it works, I recommend that you don't follow the American tradition of "If one dose is good, two doses are better." Use it in moderation.

**THE GRAIN OF TRUTH:** Flaxseed is a good natural remedy for constipation because of its high mucilage content. It's a source of fiber,
therefore, it may relieve the bloating and constipation many women
suffer prior to menstruation. Remember to drink lots of water if you
take it.

## Chasteberry (Vitex Agnus-castus)

Chasteberry is said to regulate hormones involved in the menstrual
cycle. It is purported to increase luteinizing hormone and inhibit the
release of follicle stimulating hormone. Supposedly, in some women
chasteberry acts like estrogen, in others like progesterone.

**THE BOTTOM LINE:** It isn't quite clear why chasteberry works as an
estrogen in some women and a progesterone in others. Your hormones are fluctuating greatly during perimenopause. This may be
repetitious, but I want to underscore this point: With birth-control
pills you turn off your own natural production. You substitute a measured amount of estrogen and progesterone, which creates a balance.
With chasteberry you are adding this here and that there, and no one
knows how much.

Your doctor can use everything he or she knows about medical science and still be hard put to quantify what your body is producing.
This is the reality of perimenopause. This is why perimenopause
seems like such a no-man's land in terms of absolute solutions. Hormones fluctuate wildly in these years: You ovulate one month and
don't ovulate again for four months. This causes a host of symptoms.
Adding a little bit of this or that to see if you feel better doesn't sound
like a great prescription for restoring balance to me.

**THE GRAIN OF TRUTH:** Remember — menopausal women know one thing: Their bodies are not creating estrogen or progesterone. It's a clearer picture than the one you have in transition. If menopausal women get something that acts like estrogen or progesterone from the chasteberry, it might in fact diminish some symptoms. But your body is in a different stage in perimenopause.

## Soy

Soy and many other beans have mild estrogenic activity thanks to phytoestrogens. Soy products include tofu, tempeh, miso, and soy cheese. Isoflavones are the compounds in soy that make it big news, since this class of phytoestrogens supposedly has an inhibiting effect on prostate and breast cancers.

**THE BOTTOM LINE:** There is a lot of variability in the soy products you buy at the market, due to difference in soy bean varieties and processing methods. How much phytoestrogen a particular food contains is still unknown. And, of course, maintaining a diet in which soy is a mainstay rather than an addition is a major undertaking. If you are in menopause and are thinking of adding what you need through a diet heavy in soy, you are the best judge as to whether or not you can eat enough of it to make a difference. Are you the type of person who can stay on a somewhat rigid diet indefinitely? Can you stay long enough and consistently enough on a diet of food you don't normally eat or enjoy? Your answers to these questions are important if you want to try to affect your symptoms through your diet. Realize also that soy is as fatty as many cuts of meat, although low in saturated fat, so unlikely to clog your arteries. Miso, one of the soy products often recommended, is a very salty condiment and high in calories.

**THE GRAIN OF TRUTH:** Hot flashes are rare in vegetarian cultures. Asian women have less breast and colon cancer than women in the U.S.A., and one theory as to why is that they consume more soy products. They also complain less about menopausal symptoms, although this may be a cultural phenomenon rather than a physical difference.

It's too early to say that soy will prove to be a miracle food that can banish the symptoms of menopause while fighting cancer. Much study is needed. Right now, science is still engaged in trying to figure out how endogenous and exogenous hormones work and what factors influence how much of the phytoestrogens in food are absorbed by the body.

Again, if you aren't yet estrogen deficient, the whole thing is a moot point, because soy isn't going to do much for a menses that lasts two weeks or a bout of insomnia caused by a lack of progesterone when you don't ovulate.

What may be more important for you at this stage is the research being done on the effects of soy products on the prevention of breast cancer. Does the phytoestrogen in soy products somehow work as an anti-estrogen in the breast? This is one theory and a subject of study at many major universities, notably Tufts University in Boston. However, keep in mind that Asian women also begin menstruation later than American women and have fewer years of exposure to estrogen as a result.

The research that will answer the questions about soy, whether it's safe, whether it helps, is going on right now. It is estimated that only about two ounces of traditional soy foods a day are needed to reap the possible benefits of their phytoestrogens. Tofu can be crumbled into spaghetti sauce or a casserole, and you'd never know it was there. It isn't going to hurt you to add some soy to your diet. It is a high-quality protein that supplies the body with essential amino acids, so it's healthy eating if nothing more. Better studies may exist by the time you reach menopause, and you may find it was worth the effort.

### Evening Primrose Oil

This oil, which is usually taken in pill form, is extracted from seeds that contain essential fatty acids, notably linoleic and gammalinolenic acid (GLA). GLA is used by the body to make prostaglandins, which are hormones that regulate a number of body functions.

Evening primrose oil is purported to be good for irritability, headaches, bloating, breast tenderness, and regulating the menstrual cycle. It is said to lower blood cholesterol levels and reduce high blood pressure. It is recommended as a treatment for eczema, multiple sclerosis, diabetes, arthritis, and hangovers. Native Americans used it as a sedative and a pain killer.

**THE BOTTOM LINE:** It slices and it dices! I've even seen evening primrose oil advertised as a way to lose weight in your sleep!

The steady buyer of evening primrose oil is usually going after the GLA it adds to the body. There are no studies that contain real evidence that GLA has a beneficial effect on multiple sclerosis, eczema, or cholesterol — studies in which a group took the medication and a group took placebos and the effects on each group were statistically quantified.

However, there is a lot of anecdotal evidence — in other words, success stories told by users — that evening primrose oil helps women's PMS symptoms.

**THE GRAIN OF TRUTH:** GLA is a type of essential fatty oil that your body does not make on its own. You can be lacking in it if there's not enough in your diet. Evening primrose oil will add it to your body.

More studies have been done on evening primrose oil than any other "natural" remedy. Some studies have shown benefits while others have not. No study has shown that it is better than any of the other remedies that exist for the medical problems it is advertised for. It is, however, well tolerated by the body. There doesn't seem to be any harm in using it.

## Licorice Root

Flavonoids have estrogen-like activity. A substance known as saponin supposedly has progesterone-like activity. Licorice root is purported to contain both. It also is supposed to be soothing to peptic ulcers and valuable as a cough medicine.

**THE BOTTOM LINE:** The licorice that you buy at a candy store is candy and not the same thing as licorice root. Licorice root is known to cause women to retain fluids. It promotes potassium loss and is ill-advised for anyone having problems with high blood pressure. Unless

I'm missing something here, this is about the opposite of what a women in perimenopause needs to be adding to her body.

**THE GRAIN OF TRUTH:** Licorice root is used in some over-the-counter cough medicines because it has anti-inflammatory properties.

## Motherwort

Taken as a tincture, motherwort is said to relieve hot flashes and night sweats. In fact, some women feel that it can stop a hot flash while it's in progress.

**THE BOTTOM LINE:** You're taking estrogen. Motherwort also can build up the endometrial lining and cause heavy bleeding. Some women get a rash from it.

**THE GRAIN OF TRUTH:** If you are searching for something to ease hot flashes, you are probably close to actual menopause. You need to discuss this with your doctor before trying motherwort.

## Hooked on Herbs? Protect Yourself with These Guidelines

Overall, the scientific evidence that would make me confident about recommending herbal remedies to my patients is lacking. But when a patient tells me she is experimenting with these remedies, I give the following advice.

- When you decide to try a botanical remedy, evaluate it impartially and scientifically, just as you should prescription drugs. This can be difficult. The literature that exists about these products is hardly impartial. Books favoring these "cures" often have the word *miracle* in the title. There are no studies to substantiate these miracles, although there are many women who feel these remedies help. You should monitor your body for effects, both positive and negative.
- Begin with one herb product, not a shelf full. When you take combinations of herbs it can be difficult to sort out which one is doing what to your body.
- Herbs and other natural remedies are not a substitute for profes-

sional medical care. An herbalist's suggestions for ameliorating symptoms should not be a substitute for a Pap smear, a mammogram, and a pelvic exam, which are about diagnosis. There is a wide gulf between having a medical diagnosis and merely going about ameliorating symptoms.

I was in a health-food store the other day when I heard a woman ask a clerk about echinacea. Also known as purple coneflower, it is the subject of many new studies, mostly to see if it can fight the common cold or boost the immune system.

"Do you have a cold?" the clerk asked, because that's what most echinacea customers are concerned with.

"No. I'm tired all the time. It's this fatigue."

"But are you sick? I mean, why echinacea?" he said.

"I was told to try echinacea and I'd feel less tired. Do you have it in a tea?"

She wasn't even interested in hearing what echinacea was all about. She was worried about her fatigue, and she wanted something now. The clerk said, "Have you gone to a doctor?" She shrugged. She said she was thinking of making an appointment.

This underscores the difference between going into a health-food store when you have a diagnosis and going to a health-food store for a cure to symptoms you have no real understanding of. I don't know what was causing this woman's fatigue, but I don't think she was wise to do some guessing about it and then decide that echinacea was the answer.

If you've gotten a diagnosis, and then you want to try an herb that has some potential to ameliorate that problem, I respect your desire to try an alternative approach. But I would warn anyone about making a diagnosis without the help of a doctor.

- If you are taking another regular medication, do research to find out if it can conflict with the herbs you want to take.
- Quality control is an issue you should take seriously when taking herbs in medicinal quantities. How and where an herb is grown, how it is processed, and how it is stored affect its strength. Buy them from a reliable source. Don't use anything that smells musty. If it upsets your stomach, that's enough of a reason to rethink it.
- Many doctors and health-care professionals have an understand-

ing of herbs and an open mind. If you are taking herbs or want to try them, don't assume your doctor won't understand. Always tell your doctor if you are taking herbs containing phytoestrogens. Don't conclude if your doctor raises his or her eyebrows that he or she is part of some conspiracy to sell you high-priced drugs. The drug most frequently prescribed by doctors in America is still aspirin.

- Among the more than 300 plants with estrogen-like activity that have been identified are such common foods as carrots, corn, apples, barley, and oats. Isoflavones are found in most fruits and vegetables. Perhaps "an apple a day" isn't such an old-fashioned idea for giving a boost to your overall health.

I repeat myself here, but don't confuse treatments for menopausal symptoms with treatments for perimenopausal symptoms. Menopause and perimenopause are two different places in the developmental cycle. Medical science is just starting to grasp this difference and to do serious research on the decade before menopause.

As perimenopause becomes "big business," you will hear more and more claims about "cures" for perimenopause. What doctors know now is that when a woman's body enters a stage of fluctuating hormones, she has three choices: She can add to what she has — and in the case of perimenopause it's progesterone, not estrogen, she may need to supplement. She can repress what her body naturally produces and supply a more steady dose with "cycle regulators." Or she can ameliorate her symptoms.

The key point is, assess where you are in your developmental cycle and don't take anything for menopause when you're not there yet. If you want to go the natural route, the next chapter offers the best current medical thinking on how to go about alleviating your symptoms through the most effective natural remedies of all — diet and exercise.

## Questions Women Ask

*I use natural products, mainly vegetables, because I think the body understands them better — it will use what it needs and discard the rest. The body wouldn't overuse tofu, for instance. Am I right?*

Your body is a series of biochemical reactions. The body doesn't *know* the way *you* know. There are plenty of examples where people have taken too many fat-soluble vitamins and made themselves sick. You can make yourself sick eating too much of anything. The body doesn't understand the way your brain does. The body can only respond to a series of biochemical messages.

If you're bleeding very irregularly or very abnormally, clearly your body, for whatever reason, is not producing the right amount of estrogen and progesterone at the right times. Your body is not taking what it needs and discarding the rest.

*There's something unnatural to me about using birth-control pills.*

If you come to me and say that there's something unnatural about cycle regulation (i.e., birth-control pills), and it's bad because it's not natural, I have to point out to you that the most natural form of cycle regulation is pregnancy and lactation. If you lived "naturally," you would have eight children and nurse them all for twelve to fifteen months. Most women entered into the realm of being "unnatural" the moment they decided to have only one or two children — and to have them when they were ready. The minute you used a diaphragm you monkeyed with nature.

One might argue, "I understand that, but I still have problems with taking synthetic pills." I don't want to split hairs. I am always looking to prescribe the lowest effective dosage for my patients. I've never bought into the American way of thinking that if one pill works, two will work better. What my patients want is what I want for them: good health. I just don't want you to confuse plant remedies with good health. They can be two very different things.

*I hate pills. Shouldn't one leave medicine or more serious conditions and use herbal remedies when possible?*

The real question here is What is medicine? Medicine is anything that has a biologic effect. Some medicines are natural, and some are synthetic. Digitalis comes from a plant. It's a medicine. Pills are just one type of delivery system for medication. If a medication has a systemic effect — in other words, it gets into the bloodstream and is picked up, therefore, by all the tissues in the body — then whether it's delivered through a pill, through a salve, or through an herbal tincture doesn't really matter. Don't believe that by taking herbal remedies you aren't taking medicine.

> *I don't see why doctors are so hung up on whether or not something has been scientifically tested. If something is an ancient remedy that has worked for thousands of years in another culture, why is a test even needed?*

With all the attention on "natural remedies" these days, it's interesting that the most frequent complaint I hear from women taking herbs and vitamins and teas to deal with their symptoms is that these don't do much of anything that they can tell. It's also interesting that the tablets marked "Ancient Remedy" are often the best sellers when research shows that across the world, people are turning away from traditional treatments in droves and embracing modern medicine.

Don't be taken in by the words *ancient* and *traditional,* as if anything that was manufactured in the last decade is no good. Modern medicine has the best record when it comes to saving lives. No research can dispute that.

> *Birth-control pills aren't doing the job. I'm still feeling terrible. Will something natural help?*

Maybe so, but it depends on what exactly is making you feel miserable. Keep in mind that there are many different birth-control-pill formulations. I would first want to diagnose whether your problem is estrogen related. If it is, a change in birth-control pills may be all that you need. It's easy to give up when you're taking medication and it doesn't work right away. But it can take a few months of fine-tuning with your doctor's help to find the best prescription for you.

> *Everything I read today is about natural remedies for menopause. There are books of soy recipes and articles on these remedies everywhere. I can't believe there's nothing to this.*

Many of those recipes are just plain healthful food that will help your husband as much as they do you. I have nothing against eating soy.

Again, the key word here is *menopause*. I wouldn't prescribe hormone replacement therapy for a perimenopausal women still making estrogen. Add more estrogen to your body, in whatever form, and you may very well add more symptoms.

# 5

# WILL YOU GAIN TEN POUNDS DURING PERIMENOPAUSE?
## The Secret to Weight Control During Transition

My patients' jaws drop when I tell them that I weighed 227 pounds in medical school. It's true.

I can remember the cafeteria at the hospital that I rotated through. Booth Memorial Hospital in Queens. My favorite lunch was a huge roast beef sandwich on a hard roll with mayonnaise. My mother always said, "Roast beef is protein. It's good for you." My idea of how to lose weight was to eat roast beef on a plate with barbecue sauce and skip the bread or the mayonnaise. That, to me, was dieting.

Then the cafeteria started posting the number of calories for each selection every day. Those little signs posted in the cafeteria line were an eye-opener. I realized I should have been having mayonnaise sandwiches without the roast beef. I had been ladling 900 calories of roast beef onto my plate. The hard roll had 130 calories and the mayonnaise about 100.

I would eat a salad, thinking, "This is nice and healthy." I put about 600 calories' worth of blue cheese dressing on it — it had to soak down to the bottom — and felt self-righteous about staying on a diet.

What I learned was this: It's calories in and calories out. There's no way around this. To lose weight, you either have to eat less or exercise more often to burn more of what you eat.

I lost my weight in three big blocks. I got down to the low 200s as a fourth-year medical student. I stayed there until I was close to thirty. Then I started to play squash. That got me to the next level.

I lost the last block in my forties, when I became a runner. I trained to run marathons. Then I started to run just for the economy of it — less time consuming than walking, more payoff. But many people find another sport that makes a difference.

The key for me was that I found I wasn't playing squash or running to lose weight. True, maybe in the beginning I was motivated to lose pounds. But then my competitiveness took over. I ran to run more miles than the week before, and I played squash to play squash better than I had the last game. I wasn't "on a diet." It changed my overall feeling of health. I had more energy for everything I did. Aches and pains and stomach upsets — I had them all, but I suddenly had a feeling of strength in my body. I could cope. Though my weight might fluctuate a few pounds now, I have never gone back to square one.

There is no doctor in America who hasn't discovered that women in their thirties and forties are avidly concerned about their weight. Studies show that 38 percent of women aged 40 to 49 and 52 percent of women aged 50 to 59 are overweight. Think about those numbers for a second. By age 50, more women are overweight than not.

What is hormonal? What is an excuse? What can you do to prevent a weight gain during the transitional years? This chapter will answer those questions.

## Is It Hormonal?

Women who gain weight in their thirties and forties complain, "I'm not eating more than I used to, and I'm constantly watching what I eat." I believe them. Bonnie, forty-five, is the mother of two children and a successful manufacturers' representative. She thinks back to the way she used to eat in her twenties and remembers, "Polishing off a medium-sized pizza for a snack while I studied at night was nothing. Double cheeseburgers, fried chicken — I ate it all and washed it down with a milkshake. Who knew about healthy eating then? My metabolism was going like a furnace, burning it all up. I never gained a pound.

"Then I reached my thirty-fifth birthday, and within a year I gained seven pounds, doing absolutely nothing different. Now if I don't want to gain weight I can probably eat one meal a day — small.

Maybe some broth for lunch or a salad with the thinnest suggestion of dressing. Otherwise I gain. It's ridiculous. Is the remainder of my life going to be a fork, a lettuce leaf, and Premarin on the side?"

Women who experience what Bonnie did want to know, "Is my weight gain hormonal? Can you give me some kind of hormones that will make me lose weight?"

Yes and no. I have seen a lot of women take hormones and complain that they gained weight. I have seen women take hormones and finally lose the pounds that they had been trying to lose for a decade. I have seen women who gained a tiny bit of weight on hormones and stopped taking them. Then they gained more weight. They come back to me and say, "I guess it wasn't the hormones."

## Is It My Metabolism?

A patient of mine who had just turned fifty was complaining about how she exercised an hour a day and took a killer ninety-minute aerobics class on Saturdays. She wasn't happy with the results. She had a little too much "here" (pointing to her stomach), and not enough "here" (pointing to her upper chest area).

I said, "Listen, at age fifty, an hour a day keeps what you have. If you want to start body sculpting, you are going to have to do more."

Rather than letting that fact depress you, look at what's happening to your body. During the time period in which a woman reaches transition, muscle mass decreases, body fat increases, and metabolism decreases. There's a debate about whether this is due to hormones or aging. Chances are that you will be out of this stage before medical research can give you a definitive answer.

One thing is certain: You can be eating the same amount you always ate and sticking to the same exercise program that got you through your thirties with no weight gain, and suddenly you gain weight. Five pounds come on, then ten. You are telling the truth when you say you aren't eating more or exercising less.

It is estimated that metabolic rates decline about 2 percent per decade for both men and women. If you don't change your eating and exercise habits, you will not be able to keep weight off as easily as you did when you were twenty or thirty. Women need fewer calories and more exercise to maintain a desirable body weight in their forties and fifties.

What raises metabolism naturally? Exercise and strength training. Muscle burns more calories than fat, whether a person is exercising or at rest. Every pound of lean tissue burns about fifteen more calories a day than a pound of fatty tissue.

The single most important thing you can do naturally to improve your overall physical and emotional health during transition is exercise. *Physical Activity and Health: A Report of the Surgeon General* is a 278-page summary of research into the benefits of being physically active. Released in July of 1996, it states unequivocally that physical activity is important for good health. Exercise is a natural preventative medicine. But it also found that more than 60 percent of Americans do not exercise regularly.

Many people associate exercise with cardiovascular health. Not just your heart, but your overall health will benefit from as little as thirty minutes of walking a day. Do more, and you benefit more.

My patients will tell you that I harp on this all the time. There's a reason: It changed my health, and it will change yours.

## Too Late to Lose Weight?

"I've been trying to lose the same twenty pounds for years," a patient recently told me. "Now that I'm out of my thirties, am I doomed?"

I wasn't, and there's no reason you should be. But exercise will be only part of the plan. My fifty-year-old patient who was exercising every day thought she could control her weight by working out. She kept a ten-day food diary and found that she was simply taking in too many calories. She needed to recognize that a healthful serving of meat was roughly the size of a deck of cards and that the large bagel she ate every day for breakfast was 400 calories. Simply bringing soup and grilled chicken to work for lunch rather than grazing out of the snack machine left her five pounds thinner in a month.

The healthiest way to lose weight is to reduce your calories and increase your exercise. The secret to permanent weight loss is to make this a lifestyle change rather than a "diet." Wanting it isn't enough.

You have to be willing to change your patterns for more than a three-week diet.

Take the first step. Moderate the amount of cheese, butter, nuts, red meat, and fried food in your diet. If you can eliminate them as much as possible, do it, but don't get into a deprivation pattern that makes you yearn for and binge on what you can't have. Simple moderation can help you feel better and stronger than you have in years.

Change is an easy thing to decide and a difficult thing to do. Like many doctors, I counsel patients about the importance of eating a balanced meal from the four food groups. This is old news but still the only real news. People nod their heads. Surprisingly few actually do it.

If it doesn't come naturally for you to eat a diet packed with vegetables, grains, and fruit the way it does for your teenage daughter, who goes "Ugh!" when you talk about fried chicken, perhaps it's because the rules were switched on us in the middle of our lives.

No one told us at seventeen that coating ourselves in a mixture of baby oil and iodine and roasting in the sun with a reflector wasn't going to turn out to be a wise thing for our skin. No one told us that a diet heavy on meat and potatoes was going to end up accumulating in pounds that would seem almost impossible to get rid of.

There's a huge psychological component for many members of the baby-boom generation when it comes to food. As one of my patients put it, "I grew up in a home where food was always in some state of being prepared. Breakfast was over and then the baking started. Then a brisket and potatoes floating in gravy went in the oven. My mother took it as an affront if you didn't eat her food. She believed the more you ate, the healthier you were. And exercise? My parents weren't exactly role models. Getting in and out of the car was it."

## A Plan That Works

When I speak to a patient who has a weight problem, I tell her, "People who don't have to think about what they eat, who simply eat when they are hungry and go through their lives weighing pretty much the same all of the time, have no idea what people like you and me go through. I was heavy most of my life. I understand what it's like."

The best advice I can give people about losing weight is the following:

1) If you need to lose twenty-five pounds and you have been twenty-five pounds overweight for the last fifteen years, don't try to lose twenty-five pounds in six months. You will gain it back. I can almost guarantee it.

Do it in stages. Lose a piece of the weight you need to lose and stay there. Stay there, if need be, for a whole year. Weight gain is often seasonal. Deal with it on a seasonal basis. Prove to yourself through the different seasons of the year that you won't gain it back. Then work on losing another piece of the weight.

Many people find they are more motivated if they concentrate on losing five pounds at a time. It's a realistic goal most people can reach. Setting out to lose twenty-five pounds can be overwhelming.

2) Don't give up everything you love to eat. No one stays for long on a diet of nothing but cabbage — unless she loves cabbage. I eat moderate amounts of foods I enjoy.

3) Slow down. Right before you sit down to eat, try the following regimen: Drink a glass or two of water. Exercise for twenty minutes. Set a small plate for your lunch or dinner. Vow to take your time eating. People who overeat usually eat quickly.

4) Go by how your clothes fit, rather than by what the scale says when you are dieting. If you're exercising, your new muscle weighs more than fat. You may show a weight gain on the scale at first. Daily weight readings can fluctuate for a number of reasons. If you ate salty Chinese food the night before, the weight gain you see on the scale is water you're retaining, not fat.

Daily weight swings make many women feel depressed, triggering the bad eating habits they're trying to get rid of. Weigh yourself only once a week on the same day to get the most accurate sense of your weight.

However, keep in mind that people who are successful at keeping weight off set a boundary for how much weight they can gain before something within them yells, "Stop!" Three pounds, five pounds on the scale tell them enough is enough. They make a renewed effort.

5) Be wary of "low-fat" foods. I've seen women gain weight on a low-fat diet. Low-fat muffins and granola can be loaded with calories. There are people who are loading themselves up with low-fat cookies and low-fat chips. Fat isn't the culprit for them; it's calories in — weight *on.*

6) An insane schedule is your biggest challenge. Make time to exercise regularly. This may mean involving your children in your exercise program. My six-year-old son, Luke, counts my sit-ups for me. Or he will sit on my abdomen as I do crunches. The added bonus of involving your children is that you teach them the lifelong habit of exercise. Teach your children that they should exercise every day too.

7) When you eat, don't do anything else. Of course you can speak with your dining partners, but don't talk on the phone, watch television, or read if you're having trouble with overeating. You need to pay attention to when you feel full, and you can't with so much distracting you.

8) Skip the super sizes. Super-size foods and special-value meals appeal to the human desire to get a bargain. Getting twice the french fries for a nickel more can be hard to resist, but the meal that will have the most value to you ultimately is the one with normal-size portions.

9) The patients I've known who have had the hardest time losing weight are those who feel the most depleted emotionally. They tell me, "This is the price I pay for being at the top of my field," or "This is what happens when you have three children under five."

When they look closely, their lives consist of work and food. They go top speed against rising demands all day. Finally, the work is put aside. There's a driving need for some form of release. They go and *eat,* thinking, "I'll do this just one time because I need to, then I'll get back on the plan tomorrow."

Sound familiar? Don't neglect your emotional needs. If feelings of depletion or emotional emptiness are driving you to food as solace, look at that squarely. Making time for yourself can be as important as exercise and cutting calories when you're on a diet, as is seeking ways to achieve pleasure other than food. A manicure, a massage, a hot bath, a conversation with someone you love, may substitute very well for a large meal. Seek help if you need to. You deserve peace of mind, health, vitality, a sense of balance — or what is it all for?

10) Ask yourself, "Am I willing?" Are you emotionally ready to do what it takes to change a lifelong pattern?

Consider two women who go on the same diet as partners. One loses ten pounds after a month and feels happier, healthier than she has in years. The other loses ten pounds, but she is hungry all the time. She doesn't like the menus. She eats junk food because she doesn't have time to prepare the required lunch or dinner. Then she skips meals the next day to make up for her lapse.

The first woman isn't loaded with extra time either, and she also thinks that the menus are boring and tedious. But she is willing. She is ready. She is prepared to leave the dinner table feeling unsatisfied at times. She isn't a better person. She's simply more mentally ready. She keeps the weight off, while her partner gains most of it back.

Being willing is more important than one might think. If losing weight were easy, everyone would be able to do it. Exercise with a partner. You can transform your workout into something stimulating by doing it with someone else.

## Maintaining Your Optimum Weight

Perhaps your weight is near where you want it to be. But it's increasingly hard to keep it there. You swing five or more pounds in a month. This is especially annoying because you see yourself as someone who has always been in good shape, who watches her diet, hasn't tasted a chocolate-chip cookie or guacamole and chips in a year, exercises even when she's tired. What is it all for?

The slowing down of metabolism that is part of aging makes you want to scream. Besides staying on your regimen, and maybe increasing it, here are some other things you should think about.

Severe salt restriction is one of the best things a woman can do for her body. Our diets are much too high in sodium. Your body only needs between 1,100 and 3,300 mg of salt a day to stay healthy. That's about one half to one and a half teaspoons.

The sodium contained in most foods that you buy in a prepared fashion or in restaurants is sufficient to cause water retention. Water retention gives multiple symptoms in different organ systems. One symptom is weight gain. Others are mood swings and headache. It causes breast tenderness. Generally, it can cause bloating or leg cramps.

It isn't easy to avoid salt. One tablespoon of soy sauce contains half a teaspoon of salt. Hot dogs, canned tuna, tomato juice, and even bran muffins contain a hefty amount of sodium. The typical tuna fish sandwich has about 1,118 mg of salt. A medium pickle has 928 mg.

What follows is the "low-salt" list I hand patients on a regular basis. It was put together by a top nutritionist: apples, apricots, asparagus, bananas, barley, blackberries, blueberries, brown rice, cherries, chicken, coffee, cucumber, eggplant, farina, grapes, green beans, green peppers, honey, maple syrup, oatmeal, onion, orange juice, peaches, peanut oil, pears, peas, pineapple, plain spaghetti, polished rice, potatoes, puffed wheat, raspberries, shredded wheat, squash, strawberries, sweet corn, sweet potatoes, tangerines, tea, tomatoes, vinegar, watermelon, whole wheat flour, zucchini.

If any of these foods are canned or processed in any other way, chances are the food is no longer low sodium. Check labels to see if salt has been added to the product.

Beyond limiting your salt intake, cut back on the fat in your diet. Choose meat that is "choice" over "prime," which has more fat. Choose white meat over dark when serving yourself turkey or chicken. The fat in your diet shouldn't be more than 25 percent of your total calories. When you shop, look at labels to see whether a product contains more than two or three grams of fat per 100 calories and avoid those that do. If you eat fast food, most restaurants will give you a chart that lists the fat content of each sandwich and side dish, allowing you to make better choices.

## Maintaining Your Flexibility

Flexibility training is going to be to the year 2000 what aerobics was to the 1980s. Those yoga stretches many of us dismissed because they didn't burn calories as quickly as the StairMaster are going to become more of an issue as we wonder, "Am I going to be able to get out of the backseat of a cab two decades from now? Will my body be flexible enough?"

How long has it been since you've really stretched? When people first get into fitness, it's generally through aerobics — running, fast walking, StairMaster, biking. Then they discover strength training — free weights, Nautilus, and Cybex machines.

What is ignored too often is flexibility. Life expectancy today for a fifty-year-old woman who doesn't already have cancer or heart disease is ninety-one. But as we grow older, cartilage, ligaments, and tendons become more rigid, which causes less flexibility. You maintain your flexibility by stretching and moving the joints through their full range of motion.

Stretching prevents injuries from other activities. It gives you supple muscles, which have a greater range of motion. Stretching helps you learn to feel tightness when it is building up in your body and teaches you how to release it. This is a bonus in the age of stress. You will find that you can carry out all of your daily activities with less stress and greater ease when you stretch regularly.

Even if you realize you have lost some of your flexibility, the right exercise can improve it by as much as 50 percent, no matter what your age. You can easily test your flexibility at home. Tape a yardstick to your carpet. Sit at the zero end and extend your legs in front of you along the yardstick, so that they align with the fifteen-inch mark. Now bend over slowly and try to touch your toes. Take your reading on the yardstick — how far can you go without straining? About sixteen inches is average.

Yoga classes or other flexibility classes are becoming more popular than ever. The Lotte Berk Method, taught in classes in many major cities and described in *The Lotte Berk Method* by Lydia Bach, is one of the best programs I've found for improving flexibility. The exercises are gathered from such disciplines as ballet, yoga, and orthopedic exercises recommended by physicians. The goal is to tone muscles, stretch muscles, and redistribute weight. The benefit Lotte Berk enthusiasts speak about most is increased energy. Exhaustion, according to the teachers of these exercises, isn't due to the fact that our lives are out of pace or we're overextending ourselves as much as that most of us live in a body out of tune with itself. Women with back problems will find exercises geared to toning weakened stomach muscles, which relieves pressure on the back. As an added bonus, stretching relieves tension and is relaxing. The method even includes exercises to improve sexual agility, comfort, and confidence.

The benefits of exercise and its self-discipline carry over into other areas of life. Adopt a regimen that you stick to, and I predict you will see your productivity in other areas of your life rise. Self-discipline becomes a way of life and a reward in itself.

## Protecting Your Bones

When you do any dieting or exercise programs during the years of perimenopause, it's essential that you take steps to protect your bones. Your body does not manufacture calcium. Any calcium you need your body must get from outside sources. Often a low-fat diet means less cheese, less milk — less calcium. If you don't have enough calcium in your diet, your system breaks down bone in order to supply calcium.

Researchers believe that estrogen protects a woman's bones by blocking the formation of osteoclasts — cells that break down bone tissue. But when estrogen production decreases sharply, as it does in menopause, bone loss speeds up an average of 2 percent a year. This can lead to osteoporosis — porous bones, easily prone to fracture.

The time to get in the calcium habit is now, years before menopause occurs. Besides, calcium helps the heart, muscles, and nerves function properly. Women also report that increasing their calcium intake makes them feel calmer.

You should aim for calcium intake of 1,500 mg per day. This may require an over-the-counter supplement in addition to dietary forms of it. Tums, an over-the-counter antacid, is virtually 100 percent calcium carbonate. Many antacids contain calcium. Just stay away from those that contain aluminum, which taken long-term can actually deplete your calcium reserves.

Skim milk and low-fat milk actually contain a little more calcium than whole milk. Fish and shellfish, broccoli, sardines, and collard and mustard greens are loaded with calcium without being high in

calories. Some mineral waters contain calcium. Calcium-enriched orange juice is an excellent choice for those who avoid dairy products.
Or try adding nonfat powdered milk to casseroles, pasta sauces,
soups, and other dishes.

Another weapon against bone thinning is weight-bearing exercise.
Bones are strengthened when they're subjected to forces they aren't
used to. Toning your bones with weights and muscle contractions can
increase bone mass in certain areas. Although exercise does not fully
substitute for estrogen, you can slow the rate of bone loss through a
challenging exercise program.

Advances are being made in the treatment of osteoporosis as more
research grants are given out to study it. A relatively new drug, Fosamax, available by prescription, has been shown to block the production of bone-destroying osteoclasts.

I discuss osteoporosis in more depth in chapter 10 and give you
details you should know if you've been prescribed Fosamax. It isn't an
easy drug to take and requires a high level of motivation. At your age,
there is no better way to beat the development of osteoporosis than
exercise and supplementing your calcium.

## Success Stories

When I meet a patient who has lost ten or more pounds during this
stage, I think, "What does she know that everyone else should
know?" This is what I've been told:

> *Traveling for work was a problem. I had to entertain clients. I*
> *quit eating industrial-size portions in restaurants every night; I*
> *met clients for coffee instead of dinner. And I keep a low-calorie*
> *snack in my briefcase. I make it a point never to leave work hun-*
> *gry or get on a plane when I'm starving.*
> *— Anna, thirty-seven, ten pounds in five months*

> *It takes real mental stamina to lose weight and keep it off after*
> *you've had two children. The turning point for me was realizing*
> *that I'm not twenty and I'm not going to diet for two days and lose*
> *five pounds. I quit telling myself I was horrible for not being able*

to lose it quickly. I rewarded myself for the slower progress I made.

    — *Simone, forty-one, fifteen pounds in one year*

When I want to graze through a bag of potato chips, I force myself to get up and brush my teeth. After that, I don't want to finish the rest of the bag. It breaks the cycle.

    — *Alexandra, thirty-seven, five pounds in six months*

Try exercising in the morning, before anyone can make an appointment with you or ask you to search under the bed for overdue library books. You can spend an entire day promising you're going to exercise "later," and then find yourself in bed wondering where the day went.

    — *Marci, forty-two, twenty-five pounds in fourteen months*

I've always been a fast eater. I've been in schools so much of my life. You get twenty minutes to swallow your lunch. By the time you buy your lunch, you have no time to eat it. I bring a low-calorie snack to eat during my morning break. At lunch I put my fork down after every bite. When you wolf things down, the signal that you're full doesn't seem to come. Slowing down has really helped.

    — *Evelyn, forty, ten pounds in twelve months*

I buy already-chopped vegetables at the salad bar, cooked chicken breasts at the deli, and fruit that is cut up and mixed. My grocery bills are up, but this is balanced against my biggest problem with dieting: time. When I'm ravenous at six o'clock and have about five minutes to eat, I grab whatever is handy. It's been worth the extra expense.

    — *Michelle, thirty-nine, seven pounds in two months*

When the waiter comes with the bread basket, wave him away. Don't even look at what's in it.

    — *Nancy, forty-five, five pounds in three months*

*I wouldn't walk away from my boyfriend in a bathing suit because I didn't want him to see me from the back. I did this walking backward thing with my hands covering my behind.*

*I put a ton of energy into camouflaging my weight problem or beating myself up about it. I was always thinking about it. I spent more energy camouflaging my thighs than actually doing what I needed to do to just lose weight.*

*It's like the old saying about banging your head against a wall — it really does feel good when you stop. I gave up on the expensive cellulite creams, which did nothing. I walked, I cut out fats, I cut out alcohol and desserts, and I ate more vegetables. It didn't seem like such a big deal once I was a week into it and realized I'd really made the decision to change. Weight loss is between the ears.*

*— Madeline, forty, twenty pounds in twelve months*

*I take stairs instead of the elevator — eight flights. I park my car half a mile away from work. I eat a low-calorie frozen entree for lunch that I heat up in the microwave. The scale said nothing new for a month. Then two pounds went. Then five. It worked this time because it wasn't complicated. I also realized I wanted to do it for me, not for someone else.*

*— Carolyn, forty-nine, ten pounds in three months*

*I had no control over the fine lines I was getting on my face, and I knew it. I didn't get the attention for my looks I got in my twenties. I missed it.*

*But then I thought, "I can still have an excellent body. I can be physically fit, develop some definition."*

*Don't let anyone tell you it's too late. I'm forty-seven, and this is the first time in my life that I've seen definition in my arms. They were always flabby. I never bought a sleeveless shirt. Maybe I'm vain, but I love it when women say, "How did you do it?" They say it in the same way they'd ask how I won the Nobel Prize or something. It keeps me motivated.*

*My husband says I look better now than when he married me.*

*He says it's like having a new woman in his bed. It's true. I'm not
that much thinner on the scale, but weight training has given a
whole new look to my body.*

  *— Meredith, forty-seven, seven pounds in six months*

## Questions Women Ask

*I've heard that being overweight can have one benefit: You have more
estrogen, naturally. Am I finally going to reap some benefit from these
extra pounds?*

Unfortunately, it doesn't work that way. Adipose tissue — that is, peripheral fat — makes a weak form of estrogen called estrone, which
has an estrogenic effect. This is why obese women are more prone to
get hyperplasia (overgrowth of endometrial cells, which is not necessarily cancer) and cancer of the uterus from this contribution of their
fat making constant unopposed estrogen. There are few positive fea-
tures, medically speaking, of being overweight, except perhaps for
slightly less osteoporosis.

*What about Fat Burners and other metabolizers? Will they help me
lose weight by charging up my metabolism or blocking fat absorption,
the way they claim?*

Unfortunately, there is still no miracle pill for weight loss. Metabolizers supposedly help the body convert food to energy more efficiently
so that you don't store it. This doesn't make much sense, because
medical science has proven that the more efficient one's body is at
converting food to energy, the less food you need. It becomes more
likely, not less likely, that the food you eat will go unused and end up
being stored as fat if you take a metabolizer.

The best metabolizer is daily exercise, which raises your metabolic
rate not only while you are exercising but for as long as two hours afterward.

*I think I've gained and lost the same twenty pounds five times. When
I hear about things like set point theory, or that you're stuck with the*

*number of fat cells you had in childhood, I start to feel like what's the
use. I was an overweight teen.*

So was I. It's true that there may be something to these theories, but
there are plenty of people who were chubby teens and are thin adults
who keep the weight off. The two most famous that come to mind are
Richard Simmons and Susan Powter. Reading about their struggles
can help you stay motivated. There's nothing better than a role model
when you are trying to lose weight after years of being frustrated.

*What about phenylpropanolamine? Does it really help people lose
weight?*

These are actually over-the-counter amphetamines. Some people do
find that they reduce their appetites. They can also increase high
blood pressure. Worse, once you stop taking these pills, the weight is
bound to creep back. In my opinion, during perimenopause women
already deal with enough free-floating anxiety. This isn't a good time
to add a stimulant to your body.

# 6

# RX FOR BLACK MOODS AND OTHER SYMPTOMS

These days there is sometimes much to feel moody about. Aging parents who are becoming frighteningly dependent. Teenagers going through the motions of emotional separation from their parents, rude one moment and clinging the next. The weariness that comes with telling your three-year-old for the fifth time why she shouldn't pull the cat's tail. The anxiety of decisions — should you work or stay home, live in the suburbs or the city, divorce or see a counselor, quit your job or apply to work in a new department?

Then comes the hormonal upheaval of the years before menopause. Some women cope with perimenopausal mood swings by doing nothing. By that I mean that they realize why it's happening, recognize the source, and knowing it's not all in their heads, they manage. But it isn't that clear-cut for a lot of women. Don't feel bad if after everything you've tried, it seems as if your well-worn coping mechanisms have disappeared. It doesn't mean you're weak.

Jacklyn, forty-four, was a woman none of her acquaintances would describe as weak. Still, she found that her mood swings were having an effect on the thing she cared about most — her successful career in advertising. She would be the first to tell you that no one lasts long in advertising without nerves of steel. Not on the top account. Not if that account is under review.

The weekly meeting was a tradition. This one was into its third hour and getting nasty. The VP pulled her claws out of the assistant account executive and whirled around to Jacklyn. She threw a sheaf of papers across the boardroom table. "You call this a first draft?" she shouted. "What is this mess?"

Jacklyn did something she had never done at work, much less in front of a room full of people. She burst into tears and left the meeting.

The episode lasted two minutes. It might have been overlooked at some other company, but in that corporate culture she would spend the next six months reestablishing her credibility.

She shook her head, remembering. "I'd gone through worse than that and never ended up in tears. It made me realize: *There's something wrong.* I wasn't myself. My resilience was gone. I had to do something about it."

What women like Jacklyn are experiencing is the loss of a feeling of steadiness or equilibrium. She'd felt touches of it for the past year. The trouble was, just as she decided she would see a doctor, it would disappear.

Her menstrual calendar revealed a history of anovulatory cycles. Although Jacklyn could have chosen to try low-dose birth-control pills to eliminate her ups and downs, she decided to try other strategies first and reassess in several months. She felt better after her visit. Just knowing what was happening to her body dispelled quite a bit of the angst. But when the mood swings continued to interfere with her life despite all of her self-help measures, she asked for that prescription. "I don't love being on medication," she told me, "but I can't afford half a month of a roller-coaster ride. I need some balance."

What do you do, however, if you are reluctant to take birth-control pills to restore a feeling of balance both emotionally and physically? This chapter discusses some of the best alternatives.

## Why So Little Is Known About Mood Swings

No one has ever died from a mood swing or sleep disturbance. That's why so little hard research is being done on the subtle symptoms that are such a big part of perimenopause. Still, this is a woman's health issue that needs to be addressed.

Money for women's health research was very late in coming and is still very low compared to that for research on men's health. It was well into the 1990s when Pat Schroeder and other female members of Congress succeeded in getting a significant amount of money appropriated for the Women's Health Initiative. Most of this money goes for breast cancer, osteoporosis, and heart disease research, as it should.

My views about mood swings are thus based on what I've observed in patients, not on hard research conducted by the government or the drug industry. I hope that will change in the coming decade, perhaps through the Women's Health Initiative or other programs that can focus more on the emotional and physical aspects of the period of transition before women reach menopause.

For now, the best advice I can give women for preventing mood swings is to take time-release vitamin $B_6$, also known as pyridoxine. It can help maintain your equilibrium. This vitamin helps both men and women. Give it to your husband or boyfriend. I take it. It takes a tiny bit off the edge — sort of a fine-tuning.

Try 200 mg of time-release $B_6$ every day for a month to see if it helps. It competes with a substance known as tryptophan for receptors in the brain and can help prevent mood swings often associated with PMS. Take pyridoxine only in the recommended dosage. More isn't better. Too much can make you feel sick.

Sometimes moodiness is related to bloating. A woman who feels bloated and uncomfortable — or frankly fat when water retention shows up as five or more pounds on the scale — often feels moody. Perimenopause may be the first time you experience the monthly bloating and weight gain your friends have dealt with for years. No one knows why this is so. Constipation can be the culprit. The movement of your intestines is affected by your sex hormones. Progesterone can slow the movement of the bowel so that the stools become small, hard, and difficult to pass. It's been said that estrogen speeds up the movement of the bowel, so if you're lacking in estrogen, you may have symptoms in your digestive tract. There isn't a lot of scientific evidence to prove either point, but there is plenty of anecdotal evidence. Women frequently complain of constipation the week before their periods followed by the "runs" when they get their period.

To combat bloating, increase your intake of fiber. High-fiber cereals and high-fiber breads are excellent ways to begin. Soups such as lentil and corn are also high in fiber. Fiber pill supplements are available, but some women actually find these constipating.

## Soothing Tender Breasts

Here's one more good reason for moodiness — your breasts hurt so much you can't find a bra that's comfortable. First, try cutting caffeine out of your diet. Breast tissue is sensitive to a category of compounds known as methyl xanthines, which includes caffeine, theophylline (found in tea), and bromides (found in chocolate). Approximately 50 percent of women have benign cystic mastitis, and this condition is a source of tender breasts. It can be alleviated somewhat through caffeine reduction as well as diminution of salt intake.

## When You Can't Sleep

Much anxiety and moodiness is dispelled by a good night's sleep. What do the experts recommend for insomnia?

1) Wake up at the same time each day. The best way to fall asleep is to get up early consistently. If you can't fall asleep, the antidote isn't getting more sleep in the morning to make up for the lack. Reset your internal clock by getting up even earlier. You will feel tired for a while, but you will see the payoff when you start to fall asleep more quickly.

2) Avoid weekend jet lag. Perhaps the most common mistake people make is to sleep late on the weekends. This is like flying across time zones. Avoid resetting your internal clock.

3) Reduce alcohol. It may put you to sleep, but it will wake you in the middle of the night and disturb the overall quality of your sleep.

4) Steer clear of hidden caffeine. You wouldn't dream of drinking coffee before bedtime, but did you know that chocolate, cola, Excedrin, cold remedies, and many common foods and beverages contain significant quantities of caffeine? Read the labels before you get an unexpected surprise.

5) Take time to practice letting go during the day. Just as the mind can become conditioned to stimulation, it can become condi-

tioned to relaxation. Take time each day to breathe deeply. Do five minutes of stretching exercises. Learn to meditate.

6) Stop the nighttime drama. Never take your laptop into bed and do your work if you're having trouble sleeping. Avoid stimulating movies, books, etc., while lying in bed. Condition your mind to see your bed as a place where you sleep, not where you figure out your business problems or your preteen's trouble in math class. Get up when you can't sleep and go to another room.

Don't argue in bed. Either agree to save the discussion for the morning or get up, turn on the lights, and work toward some closure. Couples who make a pact to never go to sleep with anger festering sleep better, even if they lose the hour it takes to come to a resolution.

7) Exercise during the day. It doesn't have to be an hour of killer aerobics. Take a walk. Get fresh air.

8) Avoid a heavy dinner. When you're going through a phase of having trouble sleeping, make your largest meal of the day lunch. Don't add digestion to your nightly tasks.

9) Develop a sleep ritual. There should be something you do every evening before sleeping that's regular and comforting. Maybe it's a hot bath. Maybe it's a few stretches. Make a routine for yourself that never varies. And keep your room cool (sixty to sixty-five degrees). Let the blankets provide the warmth.

10) Be realistic about sleep. Many people wake up during the night two or three times. This doesn't necessarily mean you have a sleep disorder. But if you wake up and agonize, "It took me so long to fall asleep, now I'll never get to sleep again," you've got trouble. The anticipation of not being able to go back to sleep keeps more people up than any other single factor.

11) Learn how to relax. Yes, you've read about relaxation techniques. Reading is passive. Being active means you see a specialist who demonstrates these techniques in front of you and makes you do them. There's a highly effective relaxation exercise that can be taught in forty-five minutes. You constrict and relax muscles in a prescribed order. It feels good, and you can practice it to the point that you can go through the whole regimen in five or ten minutes and benefit from it whenever you feel tense.

12) Deal with what's keeping you awake. Sometimes sleep problems are seasonal. They have to do with the absence of light during the day— a fact of life during winter. Some people find the months around the time we move the clock back or forward particularly difficult.

But often there's something on your mind that makes it difficult to let go. Are you logical, driven, perfectionist, feeling whatever you do is never enough? If this describes you, your sleep problems may be signaling more than the fact that the traffic outside your window is noisy. You've gotten out of touch with your body and its signals. You are fighting your real feelings all day and the battle is heating up at night. What's unresolved is difficult to let go.

13) Try melatonin. Many people who regularly fly across time zones swear by melatonin. Melatonin is a hormone secreted by the pineal gland, a small gland behind the eyes. The pineal gland helps regulate the sleep-wake cycle. Sometime around the age of forty-five our natural levels of melatonin decrease. People who take melatonin supplements in the form of tablets, capsules, or lozenges say that it helps them get to sleep and that they do not feel hungover or sluggish the next day, as one would from sleeping pills.

Melatonin should be taken half an hour before bedtime and works better if it's not taken on a full stomach. If you are under forty, I don't recommend it, because your body is still making all the melatonin you need. Despite the recent popularity of melatonin and the many claims that beyond helping you sleep it can prevent aging, there are no conclusive studies that guarantee long-term positive effects. Short-term use to get you back into a regular sleep-wake cycle, however, is probably harmless. Try the lowest dose first and give it a number of days to see how it affects you. Avoid it altogether, however, if you are pregnant or trying to conceive, if you have severe allergies, if you are taking steroids or have an autoimmune disease, leukemia, or lymphoma. Remember that this substance is not regulated by the FDA for purity.

14) Develop an attitude of not caring. Trying to fall asleep is a paradox. The harder you try, the more difficult sleep will become. Sleep is about letting go. Say to yourself, "It really doesn't matter if I fall asleep. My body will get enough rest just lying still." It's true.

## What to Do About Free-Floating Anxiety

Free-floating anxiety is one of the most annoying symptoms women suffering from the effects of fluctuating levels of unopposed estrogen face. It is also a problem for women in menopause. One new finding is that stable estrogen levels prevent anxiety, and that women who stop making estrogen undergo withdrawal from a natural tranquilizer.

Though Xanax, a mild tranquilizer, and Paxil, an antidepressant, are no more "natural" remedies than Loestrin, they are widely prescribed, and my patients often ask about them.

Let's take a closer look at how these drugs can be useful, their limitations, and what you should consider if they are prescribed for you.

### The Differences Between Xanax, Librium, Klonopin, Ativan, and Valium

All of these drugs fall into a category called benzodiazepines. Valium, Librium, and Klonopin are long acting; Xanax and Ativan are short acting. The long-acting benzodiazepines remain in the body days after the last pill is swallowed. The short-acting ones are out of the body a few hours after they are consumed. A long-acting tranquilizer may give you a tranquilizing effect throughout the day. The short-acting ones wear off in several hours. None of these drugs in small doses will give you the zombielike effect you may have seen in movies. Generally, they gently dispel the jitters, usually within an hour.

Some women do report drowsiness as a side effect, however. That sleepy feeling may go away after several weeks on the drug, but count on an adjustment period during which you may find yourself yawning throughout the day and in bed by eight o'clock.

Although these drugs ameliorate anxiety, they do not remove the source of anxiety, which is one reason many patients find it is difficult to go off of them. Some experience months of success and relief while taking them, but become anxious or sleepless when they try to go without tranquilizers. This is known as "withdrawal." For people taking low doses, this isn't the acute medical condition of withdrawal from substance abuse portrayed in movies. Some patients describe it as the type of moodiness you get when you try to cut out coffee when your body craves it. Others have a rebound of the anxiety they first took the drugs to dispel. It is important to avoid stopping this medication abruptly and instead taper off over several weeks. Much depends on the dose you've been taking and the drug you've been prescribed.

### Is There Anything I Can Take That's Over the Counter?

Some women swear by over-the-counter antihistamines to combat free-floating anxiety. Half a tablet of a cold remedy calms them, possibly because these drugs cause drowsiness.

### What Can I Do That's Entirely Natural to Calm Myself When I Am Feeling Anxious?

What you tell yourself when you begin to experience anxiety is crucial. You can throw yourself into a state of even higher anxiety by telling yourself that you're losing control or worse.

Doctors who specialize in panic often hear patients say, "I feel like I'm going to lose it." Some doctors encourage them. "Go ahead. You're safe here. Lose it. Give in to your anxiety." But the patients can't. Perhaps it's the permission that allays the anxiety. But the fear of "losing one's mind" is often more anxiety provoking than the likelihood that this would ever happen or the probability that it could.

Anxiety is uncomfortable, but people do not die from it. Repeat to yourself: *It's only anxiety. I can handle this. It will pass. It's not dangerous. I've gotten through this before.*

The progressive relaxation technique you can read about in detail in *The Anxiety and Phobia Workbook* is one many psychotherapists recommend to patients. With a little practice, it can help you reduce anxiety in less than three minutes. Here's how to do it:

Tighten your fists. Hold for ten seconds and then release. . . . Next, tighten your biceps by making a muscle with both arms. Hold for ten seconds and release. . . . Tighten the muscles around your eyes by clenching them tightly shut. Hold for ten seconds and release. . . . Tighten your forehead muscles by raising your eyebrows as high as you can. Hold ten seconds and release. . . . Tighten your shoulders by raising them as if you were going to touch your ears. Hold ten seconds and release. . . . Tighten the muscles around your shoulder blades by pushing your shoulder blades back. Hold for ten seconds and release. . . . Repeat as necessary. It is also important to note that walking is a better exercise than running when you're feeling anxious. Sometimes the deep breathing, or the out-of-breath feeling and the rapid heartbeat runners get, can cause anxiety. Easy does it with aerobics too on days when you're feeling jittery. A long walk at a decent pace is still terrific exercise.

## The Blue Moods

There is no medical evidence that women in perimenopause will encounter depression as a side effect. But that doesn't mean I don't hear this complaint at least once a day in my office. Beyond a regime of low-dose birth-control pills, which can help, what else can you do?

1) Exercise regularly. It's difficult to do this when you are feeling down, but it will make you feel better. Exercise relaxes, reduces stress, and increases brain endorphins, all of which can make you feel better. Anything that makes you feel better physically is going to improve your mood.

2) Recognize that you are not alone — most women have feelings about the changes before the change. When I tell patients that they are coming off their reproductive cycles, even though they might not want any more children, some find this reality uncomfortable.

In 1850 the average age of menopause was forty-six and life expectancy was fifty. Today a fifty-year-old woman who doesn't have heart disease or cancer has a life expectancy of ninety-one. And it's not coronary artery bypass and hip replacement that have people living to be ninety-one, although that may account for why they live from eighty-five to ninety-one. People are living longer because of such basic advances as water purification systems, antibiotics, vaccinations, and other technology. Men and women can feel depressed about the fact that they are getting older. But think for a moment. What's the alternative?

"We're all thinking about what's happening to our bodies and what's happening to our faces," a patient told me. "There are a lot of decisions you can't go back on that have to do with career and children. It's sad to say good-bye to that period in your life. It's not so much about not being able to have kids anymore. For most of us, we're past that. But we're saying good-bye to lots of things that regular menstruation is symbolic of."

Remember that the uncomfortable changes happening to your body during perimenopause are time limited. It's a passage you will undoubtedly make it through. You don't have a disease. You are and always were much more than your reproductive capacity.

3) Ask yourself: What's really missing? Carl Jung said that life should be divided into halves: the first devoted to forming the ego and getting established in the world, the second to finding a larger meaning for all of that effort. One is forced in midlife to look at dreams and goals and reassess them. It's a natural part of the life cycle.

You may find that you feel stalled or underappreciated. For some people, chronic low-grade depression is a retreat from feelings of anger, hurt, or sadness that arise during this time of reassessment. They try to cope with these feelings, fail to find an answer, and end up thinking, "What's the use? It's better to be numb."

Be empathetic with yourself. Your life has changed. You've grown. You've accomplished. The thought of "*What next? What now?*" needn't be depressing. It can be a creative thought.

You can begin to think of future opportunities. What can be positive about this new change in your life? What would you do right now if you knew you couldn't fail? What skills, what interests once fascinated you? What can you develop in yourself?

4) Don't grow so accustomed to feeling chronically depressed that you don't recognize it as a problem. We all experience bad moods from time to time. I feel depressed at times, and I don't make estrogen. But a loss of interest and pleasure in all your activities that doesn't pass is not something you have to live with. There is a medical term for lingering feelings of unhappiness that appear to have no known cause. The term is "dysthymia." Dysthymia is a chronic low-grade depression that affects an estimated eight million Americans.

What causes dysthymia? Some researchers believe it's a deficiency of neurotransmitters or brain hormones such as serotonin. (I'll explain this in detail in the section on Paxil and other antidepressants.)

Estrogen has been found to affect these neurotransmitters, and the relationship between shifting levels of estrogen and mood are just now being studied in earnest.

There are others who believe that dysthymia results from a psychological imbalance in thinking — a distortion in the way we perceive the events in our lives that leads to a habit of negative thoughts.

Saint-John's-wort is an herbal remedy that has been studied for its success in treating dysthymia. It is available at health-food stores and some drugstores. The manufacturers say it nutritionally supports a feeling of well-being. Widely used throughout Europe to combat depression, it is becoming quite popular in the United States. One capsule is taken three times a day. Generally, people experience some relief in three weeks.

## Progesterone and Depression
The crankiness that some women experience the week before menstruation has long been attributed to progesterone. Changes in the stimulation of progesterone receptors in the brain, it is theorized, can bring on bad moods.

But progesterone, whether it is naturally occurring or a part of hormone replacement therapy or birth-control pills, is something women need. It protects the uterus from cancer and balances the symptoms of estrogen. Sometimes just knowing that progesterone is the reason you feel a little off, a little less inclined to be pleasant, is enough. A different brand of birth-control pills or HRT progesterone supplements may help.

## Paxil, Other Antidepressants, and PMS
Chances are that you have read or heard about Paxil as a "high-tech" treatment for premenstrual moodiness. It's receiving a lot of media coverage as a panacea for "hormonal problems." Paxil, along with Prozac, Zoloft, and Serzone, are antidepressant medications known as "serotonin reuptake inhibitors."

Your brain has a natural level of certain neurotransmitters, one of which is serotonin. The brain breaks down serotonin as a natural process. It is hypothesized that in some people the brain breaks down the serotonin too quickly, causing a depressed feeling. Antidepressants such as Paxil balance the supply of naturally produced neurotransmitters by inhibiting their reuptake, thus keeping them around in greater quantity. When you take a drug such as Paxil you are not adding "synthetic" serotonin but trying to hang on a little longer to what you already have. This is why many psychiatrists refer to such drugs as a "natural" treatment for depression.

Many women are prescribed Paxil or Zoloft because they complain of low energy, fatigue, or just not feeling themselves. These symptoms can be interpreted as depression and sometimes go along with true depression. But the symptom of low energy is often hormonal.

There have been studies on lab animals that show some indication that a drop in estrogen may cause a corresponding drop in serotonin, which could help explain women's mood swings and feelings of anxiety and irritability.

Antidepressants are not painkillers or tranquilizers. You do not generally "feel" them in the way you would those drugs. What are they like? One patient told me that after she started taking Paxil, she kept looking for a change in herself, but it wasn't immediate.

"It's not a happy pill. You don't get high from it. It hasn't done much about the very vivid, mind-numbing depression I get a day before my period. I don't think I would have tried something like this just for my PMS, because it's an expensive regimen and you have to constantly see the doctor.

"My mouth is dry a lot and I'm more tired. But I'm feeling steady where I once felt lost. I feel much better. I feel that I'm becoming not someone else but more myself."

## Menstrual Migraines

The one-sided aching along with the nausea, vomiting, and sensitivity to light that characterize migraine headaches are scary if you haven't experienced them before perimenopause. The reason these headaches occur at this time of your life most probably has to do with fluctuating estrogen levels, especially when the estrogen level drops after a period of being high.

Drugs that constrict the blood vessels in the brain can help banish preperiod migraines. One commonly prescribed drug is Bellergal, which is also a tranquilizer. There are many other drugs your doctor may recommend. You often need to take Compazine, an antinausea medication, along with them, because these drugs can cause nausea and vomiting.

Premenstrual migraines are no laughing matter. If they are frequent and incapacitating but you don't wish to take medication, you need to think carefully about anything that might trigger them beyond menstruation. Alcohol and chocolate are mentioned by many women as possible triggers. Limiting caffeine may also help.

## Crushing Cramps

Cramps cause moodiness as well as physical discomfort. There isn't much you can do about the fact that your body produces prostaglandins just before your period. In some women, these prostaglandins cause uterine contractions that are painful and cause crushing cramps. Oral contraceptives, which stop ovulation, will lessen this flow of prostaglandins but won't eliminate them completely. Beyond that, aspirin or Motrin (one brand of ibuprofen — there are others) can be helpful. Breathing exercises, like those they teach women in Lamaze classes to ride out the contractions of labor, can be helpful in managing cramps.

## Forgetfulness — Is There Anything You Can Do to Increase Your Mental Fitness?

Researchers say there may be a link between mental acuity and estrogen level. The brain, like the uterus and breasts, contains estrogen receptors, sites where hormones affect cells. New research proposes that estrogen receptors influence function in the part of the brain called the hippocampus, which is mainly responsible for memory. There is strong evidence that the hippocampus's ability to store information changes during the menstrual cycle. A drop in estrogen, even a temporary one with fluctuation, it's hypothesized, may temporarily reduce the number of connections between neurons — brain cells through which signals are transmitted — leading to an inability to concentrate and forgetfulness. You may therefore have different levels of memory at different times in your menstrual cycle, according to these findings.

The memory lapses you sometimes experience, where you can't remember your fax number or the street the dry cleaner is on, while alarming, are normal and are related to fluctuating levels of estrogen during perimenopause.

To help your memory, you may find it necessary to exercise your brain as much as your body at this point. Here are some tips that may help.

1) Summarize. If you've been listening to a speaker, watching a program, or reading a book, stop occasionally to summarize the main points to yourself.

2) Use picture clues. To memorize names, for example, conjure up some mental pictures. You meet a man named Mike McElligot, so you picture an elegant McDonald's. For Ray Tyler, imagine a big necktie with pictures of the rays of the sun on it. This was a trick taught in the famed Dale Carnegie "How to Make Friends and Influence People" seminars. You can also create a silly story to help you remember a list of items.

3) Record reminders for yourself. Pocket-size recorders can be found for about twenty dollars at electronics stores. They are about the same size as a small calculator. Press a button, speak, and your message is recorded for you. You can record quite a few messages, and you can erase the ones you don't want to keep without disturbing the rest, no matter what order you recorded them in.

4) Reduce your stress. Anxiety saps memory. So does sleeplessness. Give your mind regular vacations through meditation. If you are a worrier, therapists recommend setting up a half hour a day as your worry time. When your thoughts start to meander to your problems, say, "Stop," and vow to wait for your worry time.

5) Use notes, highlighters, and a day planner. Always take paper and a pen with you when you leave the house, and keep them in your car as well.

6) Repeat things you need to remember to yourself immediately. Say them aloud. If you're introduced to someone new, use the person's name in your next sentence.

## Questions Women Ask

*Is compulsive eating a symptom of perimenopause?*

Many women report increased appetite before their period at all ages. Generally this is part of premenstrual syndrome, which may get worse as your hormone levels begin to change.

*This might sound strange, but I'm becoming accident prone. Could that have anything to do with perimenopause?*

Clumsiness has often been reported as a symptom of PMS, as women become more distracted. That bloated, ungainly feeling may also contribute to this. If you're feeling worried and anxious and it's difficult to concentrate, you may in fact become accident prone.

*I feel tired and sometimes dizzy around the time of my period. Is there anything I can do about this?*

Sometimes this is caused by the eating binge that some women experience right before they menstruate. These women tend to crave sugar and fill up on sweets. Their blood sugar drops abruptly several hours later, and they feel tired, dizzy, and nauseous.

Try eating foods high in complex carbohydrates and proteins. Whole grains, fish, fresh fruit, and fresh vegetables all take longer than other foods to be converted into glucose by your body. This may help to keep your blood-sugar level more stable. Also, avoid caffeine and alcohol. If the situation doesn't improve with these measures, have a discussion with your doctor.

# 7

# HOW TO STAY OUT OF THE O.R.

Abnormal bleeding is one of the chief complaints that bring women into the gynecologist's office. Until recently, if these women were past thirty-five, most of them were headed for the operating room. Every day in this country hundreds of women undergo dilation and curettage (D&C) for diagnosis when they could have a simple, painless procedure in their doctors' offices instead.

This chapter highlights a state-of-the-art technique — sonohysterography — that I use to eliminate the need for diagnostic surgery in potentially three-fourths of cases of abnormal bleeding. Armed with this knowledge, any woman can avoid an unecessary trip to the O.R.

## A Troubling Diagnosis

Recently, the nurse in day surgery said to me, "Dr. Goldstein, why is it all your patients have something?"

I asked what she meant. She said, "Well, the patient Tuesday had a polyp, and the week before the patient had a fibroid, but they always have something. Other doctors bring patients to day surgery, and sometimes they have something, but just as often they don't."

I explained to her that in my hands, the patients who have "nothing" never come to the O.R.

Cindy, forty-six, is a case in point. She was told by her doctor that she needed a D&C to find out the cause of her abnormal bleeding. "When my period came, there was no question something was wrong," she recalled. "I was going through a pad every hour. I ruined two pairs of pants."

But did she need surgery to find out the cause? "My mother had two D&Cs, so I thought it was no big deal. Then the nurse came in and started grilling me about insurance. All of a sudden it hit me that a D&C is surgery. It means anesthesia. A trip to the operating room. A hospital stay. Days off from work. Someone to watch my kids. Insurance nightmares.

"I was sorry I even mentioned the bleeding. It didn't seem that bad all of a sudden. We had enough financial problems. Did I really need all of this?"

Although Cindy's doctor recommended surgery, sometimes the most distressing diagnosis a patient hears is "Don't worry about it; the problem will go away by itself."

Since her second child, Shari, thirty-eight, had had extremely heavy bleeding and cramping. Her OB-GYN told her to wait, that it would go away by itself. "But it didn't stop, and it didn't get better. When you bleed that heavily, your first thought is 'What if this means cancer?' How long can you go through something like that and not worry?

"I had two preschool kids. I couldn't take a day off when the cramps got so bad I couldn't stand up straight. I'd force myself to get out of bed. There were days when I'd lie on the couch curled up in a ball while my husband stared and the kids dined on McDonald's. He didn't think this was normal either.

"I wasn't looking for surgery, believe me. But I was looking for a doctor who would take my symptoms seriously. I was sick of all of this bleeding. It wasn't normal to be in this much pain, and I knew it."

Cindy's problem was a hormonal imbalance, which responded to medication. She never went to the O.R. Shari's cramping and bleeding was caused by a polyp, which her uterus was trying to expel. The polyp was removed, leaving her symptom free.

I diagnosed both women without a D&C, although Shari eventually needed one for therapy — *not* for diagnosis. The difference between having a D&C for diagnosis and for therapy is crucial.

A new procedure that can be done in virtually any gynecologist's office with a high-quality ultrasound machine can eliminate the need for diagnostic D&Cs. Women whose bleeding is hormonal don't need D&Cs at all. Those women whose bleeding is caused by polyps, fibroids, precancers, or even cancers need surgery for therapy.

## What Exactly Is a D&C?

D&C stands for dilation and curettage, a procedure in which doctors dilate the cervix and then scrape the endometrial lining of the uterus. The procedure has been around since 1843. It's done both for diagnosis — to find out why a woman is bleeding abnormally — and therapeutically, and to remove certain growths in the uterus.

It's the most common surgical procedure women undergo in America. They are told it is a routine procedure. But it is still surgery — requiring anesthesia and the risks that go with it. Worse, three-fourths of these invasive and costly operations are unnecessary: They turn up nothing.

In a study I recently headed, 79 percent of perimenopausal patients with abnormal bleeding had no anatomic abnormalities. They simply had a hormonal imbalance (lack of ovulation, or "dysfunctional uterine bleeding," in medical jargon).

## What Is the Most Frequent Cause of Heavy Bleeding?

You can have very heavy, very scary bleeding from nothing more than a hormonal imbalance. Without progesterone, unopposed estrogen in your system may cause heavy, clotty bleeding that is different from the menstrual periods you've experienced before.

It is also true that you can have abnormal bleeding — heavy or at the wrong time or both — from cancer, hyperplasia (precancer), polyps, or fibroids. The key to staying out of the O.R. is knowing what's wrong before you are automatically given surgical treatment.

## Why Do So Many Doctors Recommend D&C?

If you are twenty-five years old and bleeding twice a month, this is invariably a hormonal imbalance (dysfunctional uterine bleeding). You are usually treated with birth-control pills or simply some reassurance about why this is happening.

If you are thirty-five with the same scenario, it is still almost always dysfunctional uterine bleeding. But if you are forty-five, modern gynecology has always felt a need to rule out any serious organic causes of bleeding (polyps, fibroids, hyperplasia, or cancer). Abnormal bleeding in this age group has thus always triggered some sort of sampling of the lining of the uterus, usually through D&C.

The problem is that the vast majority of D&Cs never turn up any abnormalities, and the bleeding is attributed to hormonal causes. Although some doctors recommend endometrial biopsy instead of D&C, it is of extremely limited value. In a recent study of 433 perimenopausal patients with abnormal uterine bleeding, it was demonstrated that an office biopsy alone would have potentially missed polyps, submucous myomas, and hyperplasia in up to eighty patients, or 18 percent of the time. That is because a biopsy, in which an instrument is passed into the uterus and a small piece of the lining removed, samples such a small area of the uterus. If the abnormality involves only a *portion* of the lining (medically known as "focal" rather than "global"), as polyps and many hyperplasias and cancers do, it is totally hit-or-miss as to whether a biopsy done blindly will reveal it.

A hysteroscopy can also be recommended. In hysteroscopy, a small fiberoptic scope is placed into the uterine cavity. Saline solution is used to expand the uterus so that the endometrial surface can be viewed. It requires general anesthesia, because the doctor needs to dilate the cervix enough to place the scope into the endometrial cavity. Some practitioners use smaller instrumentation to do office hysteroscopy without general anesthesia. They claim it is not painful, although most patients agree that it is uncomfortable even with local anesthesia.

Vaginal probe ultrasound and fluid-enhanced sonohysterography can eliminate the need for almost all diagnostic D&Cs, hysteroscopy, and blind endometrial biopsies. Thousands of doctors across the country are now embracing these techniques.

Sonohysterography came into general use in 1994. It is a procedure whereby a small amount of sterile saline solution is put into the uterine cavity through a tiny plastic catheter. (One model many doctors use is known as the Goldstein catheter, which I developed. It looks like a piece of uncooked spaghetti.) The vaginal ultrasound exam is then conducted while saline is being infused.

The procedure is absolutely painless, takes a few moments to perform, and can be done by virtually any OB-GYN who has ultrasound equipment. Current estimates are that upwards of 75 percent of OB-GYN offices have ultrasound equipment.

The detail is phenomenal: A doctor can see the uterine lining almost as if he or she were looking at it under a low-power microscope. If nothing turns up on the sonogram, no surgery is necessary. If the sonogram finds something, the doctor knows what to expect in surgery, so the right personnel and equipment are available, depending on whether there is a polyp, a fibroid, or something else.

Study the simple ultrasound pictures that appear in the Appendix. You can clearly distinguish between a uterus with "no anatomic abnormality" typical of dysfunctional uterine bleeding and those with polyps, fibroids, or thickened focal tissue suggestive of precancer or cancer.

## What Should You Ask if Your Doctor Says You Need a D&C?

If you are told by your doctor that you need a D&C, your first question should be *why?*

Your doctor may answer, "Well, I want to make sure there is nothing bad going on."

Ask, "What does *something bad* mean? What are the chances that this is just hormonal? And if it could be hormonal, are there any simpler, cheaper, less invasive ways, such as ultrasound or fluid-enhanced ultrasound, to determine that I don't have a fibroid, polyp, precancer, etc., without first having a D&C?"

You might also ask: "Can I give it more time to see if the problem clears up on its own? What are the risks if I decide to go without treatment at this time? Can this problem be helped with medication?"

If you are satisfied that you truly need a D&C, the most important question you need to ask concerns hysteroscopy, which I described earlier in this chapter. A hysteroscopy should be a part of the D&C. Here's why it is so important:

Dilation and curettage is a procedure that was — and often still is — done blindly. The cervix is dilated so that an instrument can be passed into the endometrial cavity, and scraping is done by feel, without the doctor seeing inside. Numerous studies have shown that as much as 50 percent of the uterine cavity goes unsampled in a blind D&C procedure. In addition, some of the newer small biopsy suction instruments sample as little as 4 percent of the endometrial surface area.

You're going into the O.R. You want the best medical science has to offer. Hysteroscopy involves putting a fiberoptic scope into the endometrial cavity so that the doctor can actually visualize its contents. From my point of view, anyone going to the O.R. to have a D&C in 1998 or beyond *must* have hysteroscopy as part of it, because a blind D&C will be fraught with error.

If you need a D&C for therapy, and hysteroscopy will be part of it, be reassured that a D&C is day surgery. You usually go in an hour before the procedure and go home an hour after. You will need to come in within a week before for presurgical testing, which includes a blood count and simple urine analysis. It also requires a taking of your medical history. This may lead to other tests. Occasionally an electrocardiogram or a chest X ray may be ordered. But for the overwhelming majority of healthy peri- and early postmenopausal patients, a simple blood test for both white and red blood counts, hematocrit, platelets, and urinalysis are sufficient.

After the surgery, you may experience a little bit of cramping, but you're basically 100 percent the next day. I tell patients that how they feel at four P.M. on the day of their D&Cs depends more on how they react to the short-acting anesthetic than on the procedure itself.

## How to Avoid an Unnecessary Hysterectomy

A hysterectomy is removal of the uterus. There are many reasons it might be appropriate for a patient. Hysterectomy for cancer is always appropriate. Endometrial cancer is the most prevalent gynecological cancer, with about 34,000 new cases a year. It is also one of the most curable. Stage one uterine cancer has a survival rate upwards of 90 percent. If it is picked up early, it is a very treatable disease.

Uterine prolapse is another problem where hysterectomy may be indicated. Prolapse occurs when the muscles and ligaments that hold the uterus in place become extremely stretched or weakened. This can occur as a result of childbirth and as you get older. Sometimes the cervix and the uterus will start to hang out of the lips of the vagina and rub against your clothes. Still, a prolapse that severe would be very, very rare in a woman at the age of perimenopause.

Unfortunately, *the most common reason women end up having hysterectomies today still has to do with abnormal bleeding.* As one patient told me, "My doctor recommended a hysterectomy after only a pelvic exam. 'You don't want more children; so see if it helps.' "

I have met hundreds of women who are frankly scared about bleeding and almost at their wits' end. But in a study I recently organized, we saw 433 women who were experiencing abnormal perimenopausal bleeding and didn't find one cancer. There were a handful of precancers. I removed fifty-six polyps in a row without one being true cancer. The incidence of frank malignancy in women of perimenopausal age is very low.

Hysterectomy is a major operation. It involves a general anesthetic. It's costly. Generally you have the surgery and go home on the third day. I've known women who go back to work after two weeks, but I can tell you that they don't go back to work feeling great. Surgery takes a lot out of a person. I advise people to count on a recovery period of up to six weeks. Hysterectomy also results in sudden menopause if the ovaries are removed, no matter what a woman's age.

Hysterectomy for cancer is a given regardless of the recovery time. But for abnormal bleeding, it should be looked at as the last resort. To understand why, let's take a closer look at three common causes of abnormal bleeding in women thirty-five and up when the bleeding is not hormonal: fibroids, polyps, and hyperplasia.

### Surgery for Fibroids? Just Say No

Kathryn, thirty-six, went to pick up the dress she'd be wearing as matron of honor at her younger sister's wedding. She had her three-year-old with her, who was cranky from missing a nap. "It's really our store policy not to let customers take a dress without a last fitting," the salesperson told Kathryn. "Try the dress on, just to be sure."

So Kathryn, crabby daughter in tow, reluctantly went into the fitting room, where she found that a dress she was supposed to wear in twenty-four hours would not zip at the waist comfortably. She could hold in her breath and squeeze it shut, but the zipper looked as if it was threatening to pop. She was tired and upset, and the idea that the store could have made a mistake like this brought a sharp edge to her voice and a request to see the manager. The salesperson whipped out a tape measure. There was no mistake. Kathryn was a half inch bigger below the waist than she had been two months ago, when she'd had her last fitting for the dress.

"Looking back, I guess it was a blessing," she says. "My stomach had been upset; I'd felt bloated. But there was no question that the lower part of my abdomen was swollen, like I'd grown this little pot belly. You might wonder why I didn't see this in the mirror, but with this wedding going on I barely had time to think. And of course, most women get bloated every now and then. I just thought it was my period."

Kathryn's abdomen was swollen from a fibroid tumor that had enlarged her uterus. It's estimated that two in five women under fifty will be diagnosed at some point in their lives with a fibroid tumor. Fibroids (also called myomas or leiomyomas) are very common in women during perimenopause. Unopposed estrogen stimulates their growth. Genetics also plays a role, as does being overweight.

One can hear the word *tumor* and feel terrified. But a fibroid tumor isn't cancer. It's a mass of muscle and connective tissue in the uterus. Fibroids arise in the wall of the uterus. If a fibroid stays within the wall, it's called intramural. If it grows into the endometrial cavity, it's called submucosal.

Fibroids range in size from as small as a pea to the size of an orange or occasionally even a basketball. But even patients with relatively large benign fibroids do not necessarily need to be operated on.

In the past, when the uterus achieved a size known as twelve weeks (about the size of a large orange), doctors often recommended the patient have the fibroid removed. Doctors felt they could no longer adequately evaluate the ovaries during a pelvic exam if the uterus was that large. The danger was that ovarian cancer could go undetected, and it was better to protect the patient.

Today, ultrasound imaging makes it possible to look closely at the ovaries despite the presence of fibroids. With the ability to visualize the ovaries using ultrasound, there is no longer an absolute size at which a fibroid must be removed.

Women with fibroids often talk about pressure symptoms. Fibroids sometimes lean on the bladder. Still, fibroids are slow growing, and the adjacent organs accommodate very nicely in the overwhelming majority of cases. In addition, if you operate for "symptoms" from fibroids, often these symptoms are not relieved. As women get older, they tend to feel the need to urinate more frequently, as do men. This is often unrelated to fibroids. It is easy and convenient to attribute any symptoms in the lower abdomen and pelvis to fibroids, but it is my experience that often these symptoms are not relieved in their entirety, or at all, with surgery.

If your fibroids are not large, not causing extreme bleeding, and not growing rapidly, it is usually fine to watch and wait. If you bleed heavily, you will want to include plenty of iron in your diet to ward off the possibility of iron-deficiency anemia. Be aware, however, that too much iron can cause constipation. Follow the instructions on the label of any over-the-counter iron supplement you buy.

The decision to opt for surgery is ultimately yours. After menopause, when estrogen levels are lower, fibroids shrink naturally. However, if you are having painful cramps or heavy menstrual bleeding, you may want to consider surgery. Consider it only after you have been thoroughly evaluated with ultrasound and possibly saline-infusion sonohysterography. Myomectomy — surgical removal of the fibroid while leaving the uterus in place — is sometimes an option. It is one possibility for women who still want to have children. However, myomectomy is usually an open operation that is every bit as complicated from a surgical point of view as a hysterectomy.

Lack of appropriate counseling and information is generally why women who don't want more children have myomectomies in the old-fashioned way, with all of the risks and recovery time involved, because they want to "keep their uteruses." My advice to such women has always been that if you are going to subject yourself to a major operation, you should do the correct operation, and that is simple hysterectomy. The cervix can be left behind, as there is still some debate about the function of the cervix in sexual activity. The ovaries can be left behind if they are still functioning. But if you have a diseased uterus to the point where you are going to have an open operation with general anesthesia, my point is to do the correct operation. If the problem is bleeding due to submucous myomas, you can opt for a resectosopic myomectomy, a whittling procedure through the cervix that is not much more involved than a D&C if the surgeon has the skill and equipment to do it.

Fibroids are the cause of abnormal bleeding in only about 5 percent of patients, whereas one-third of women have fibroids. Thus, in the overwhelming majority of women with fibroids, abnormal bleeding is the result of the hormone imbalance (dysfunctional bleeding) I have previously described. It can make good medical sense not to operate but to treat those patients hormonally. If the fibroids coexist with the dysfunctional bleeding, the treatment is hormonal. If the fibroids are submucous and the *cause* of the bleeding, then the fibroids are treated.

## When a Polyp Is Causing Your Bleeding

A polyp, technically speaking, is a tumor, although it's almost always a benign tumor. Generally, polyps are harmless.

A polyp is a growth with its own central blood vessel, as opposed to tissue growth. The bigger ones I've seen range from the size of a thumbnail to the size of a lime. Polyps have a connection to the uterine lining known as a stalk. Sometimes the stalk is very broad, sometimes very narrow. But whatever their appearance, they are growths derived from endometrial tissue projecting into the endometrial cavity. Polyps can be a major source of abnormal bleeding. Sometimes they cause cramps as the uterus tries to expel them.

Since a polyp is inside of the uterus, your doctor can't feel it during a pelvic exam. In the past, the only way to diagnose a polyp was to do a D&C.

With ultrasound a doctor can see the lining of the uterus. Let's say the lining looks thick in an area. The thickness might be a polyp off the front wall, for example. However, since the uterus is collapsed, the doctor can't really be sure. With saline-infusion sonohysterography, fluid can be introduced into the uterus, which slightly separates the front and back walls from each other. Now the doctor can clearly see the difference between an abnormality that is focal, meaning coming off just one area, like a polyp, versus abnormal buildup of tissue, which occurs in every nook and cranny of the endometrium and is known medically "global."

Once a polyp is removed (during a D&C or hysteroscopy), it is not likely to recur. Still, have the D&C only to remove the polyp you already know about, not to find out if you have one or not.

### Understanding Hyperplasia

Hyperplasia is increased growth of tissue that is abnormal. There are different types of hyperplasias of the endometrium. Some of them are precancerous, and some are not.

If you have hyperplasia, it can be removed, but if you don't do something about what's causing it, it is just going to grow back. Much of hyperplasia is related to unopposed estrogen and needs to be treated hormonally, usually with generous doses of progestins.

## Cancer Fears and Realities in the Year 2000

Heavy bleeding episodes can be scary. Many of my patients fear cancer immediately. However, the fact is that if you are a woman in your thirties or forties entering the transitional time prior to menopause, you are statistically not a high risk for any of the gynecological cancers.

The untimely death of Gilda Radner from ovarian cancer and her husband Gene Wilder's relentless public relations campaign did a tremendous amount to enhance the awareness — and the anxiety — of the American public about ovarian cancer. If you have no family history of ovarian cancer, your chances of getting it at all are low — 1.4 percent. Your chances of being diagnosed with it now, in perimenopause, are even lower. Eighty percent of ovarian cancers involve women over fifty.

If you are at risk for ovarian cancer, your best safeguard is probably an ultrasound-enhanced bimanual exam with visualization of your ovaries twice a year.

Ovarian cancer isn't the death sentence it used to be. I have removed ovaries in women with very early cancer tissue and they have gone on to have children and live their lives much as they did before.

## Breast Cancer Myths and Realities

My patients dread breast cancer, and it's certainly understandable, but women who have not reached menopause often seriously overestimate their risk. There are three myths about breast cancer I'd like to dispel.

### Myth #1: You have a one in nine chance of getting breast cancer today

Women do indeed have a one in nine chance of getting breast cancer over their entire lifetime. But that is *if they live to age ninety.* You have to live past the average life expectancy. You have to avoid heart disease. The statistic for succumbing to heart disease by age ninety is one in two!

According to the American Cancer Society, your risk of developing breast cancer by age 35 is 1 in 600; by age 40, 1 in 212; by age 45, 1 in 93; by age 50, 1 in 49.

By the time your risk factor becomes one in nine, there may be medical advances that offer a cure. You have your youth on your side. By the time you read this, new medications may be available (see chapter 11 on raloxifene). Research shows that the death rate for breast cancer is currently slowly descending. And increased cases of breast cancer may have more to do with the fact that women are going to the doctor and getting mammograms and detecting the disease early than anything else.

### Myth #2: If you have many of the risk factors, you will probably get breast cancer, and there's nothing you can do about it

The risk factors for breast cancer most doctors agree on include having had a female relative diagnosed with the disease, early menstruation (before age twelve), late menopause (after fifty-five), having no children or the first child after thirty, heavy alcohol consumption, and obesity. But there are studies that show that most women with these known risk factors never develop the disease. More than 80 percent of breast cancers are diagnosed in women who have no history of it in their families.

Every woman can take steps today to cut her risk of developing breast cancer. Cut your fat intake. Limit your alcohol intake to no more than two drinks per day.

Early detection isn't the same as prevention, but it's the next best thing medical science offers. Have a mammogram at age forty to have a baseline against which a doctor can measure future changes. Then have one every other year until age fifty, when I recommend having the test annually. (I give tips on how women can get the most out of a mammogram in chapter 8.) Examine your breasts regularly, and if you don't, admit this to your doctor. Sometimes a simple office lesson in conducting a self-exam will demystify the whole procedure.

## Myth #3: Breast cancer means losing a breast

A woman I met after a lecture recently told me this story: "My mother died of breast cancer. It was terrible to watch. Her breast was removed, and she made it past the five-year mark. We thought she was in the clear. Then she was diagnosed again.

"I go for regular mammograms and do my own exams. But my sister refuses to see a doctor. She refuses to do anything that has to do with medicine and spends her time in health-food stores, going on diets that are supposed to detoxify her body. She figures why go to a doctor if you can't do anything about breast cancer anyway."

True, doctors don't win every time in the battle against breast cancer. But they are winning more and more often today with early detection. Unfortunately, massive publicity geared to helping women learn more about breast cancer so they can avoid it or treat it makes many women feel vulnerable. The reality of breast cancer is this: If you catch it in its early stages, a lumpectomy may be all you need. We have the medical technology to help you catch it. In every case, early detection gives you more options.

Regular doctor appointments, an honest dialogue about your

fears, a healthy lifestyle — this is where you aim if you want to minimize your chances of breast cancer. This is what reduces your odds of health problems and enhances your chances of recovery should symptoms appear.

## Questions Women Ask

*What is "endometrial ablation"? My doctor suggested this as a remedy for my very heavy bleeding.*

Endometrial ablation is a form of burning or coagulating or cauterizing or just destroying the uterine lining tissue with an electric current or heat so there's nothing there to bleed. The tissue scars over and will no longer respond to hormones. In effect, it cuts the bleeding significantly or almost totally.

The problem I have with this procedure is that once I eliminate all the possible causes of bleeding, like polyps, hormonal problems, precancers, and fibroids, I can't find too many women who need endometrial ablation.

If you're sick and tired of bleeding, and your doctor can't find anything the matter, he or she may well suggest this procedure. In my opinion, depending on the specifics of your case, you might be far better off taking Loestrin or another low-dose birth-control pill. If your doctor can't find anything wrong, and you continue to have bleeding, the overwhelming likelihood is that the bleeding is in fact dysfunctional uterine bleeding. Rather than undergo a surgical procedure to try to burn the lining of the uterus in the hopes that it scars and therefore will no longer bleed, you would be far better off trying cycle regulation with a low-dose birth-control pill to see if it will control the bleeding without surgery, anesthesia, expense, and discomfort.

*Why are you so against D&Cs? My mother had one, and it took care of her bleeding. My doctor believes a D&C is no big deal.*

I'm not against D&Cs for therapy, but for the past fifty years D&Cs have been the gold standard for diagnosis. More recently many practitioners have added hysteroscopy to the regimen. My feeling is simply that now there is a better way. Ultrasound and saline-infused sonohysterography can give doctors as much information in a safer and painless office procedure.

A sonohystogram can be done at the time of the pelvic exam. You don't feel anything painful, and in about as long as it takes to have a regular exam, you're done. No scheduling surgery, thinking, "I've got to take a day off, my husband's got to come pick me up, someone has to take care of my kids, I've got to come in for presurgical testing. Is my insurance going to cover it? Am I going to have a complication? What's going to happen? What are they going to find?"

As for your mother, she may not have had any other options. D&C used to be the most common operation in America. Saline-infusion sonohysterography is state-of-the-art, a child of technology newly available in this decade.

*Both my mother and grandmother had hysterectomies. Does this*
*mean I will be more likely to eventually need one too?*
Many baby boomers' mothers or grandmothers had hysterectomies. One of my patients recalls her mother being told by her doctor, "We're going to remove the cradle but leave the playpen."

It's a well-researched fact that more than half of those hysterectomies could have been avoided. Many of those women endured an operation to remove a uterus that was healthy. Worse, after they went through all that, whatever their symptoms were, they remained.

When you can avoid major surgery, do it. I don't want to scare people, but there are risks of major surgery related to both the anesthesia and the surgery itself. With anesthesia, a tube has to be put in your windpipe, and you have to be ventilated by machine for the two hours that the operation takes. There is a small but real risk of the tube's not being positioned properly for adequate ventilation and oxygen profusion. You can have lung complications. There can be damage at the time of surgery to the urinary or gastrointestinal tracts resulting in the need for subsequent operations, or there is the possibility of fistula formation, where patients can lose urine though the vagina. Postoperatively, people can be prone to pneumonia, to infection, to hemorrhage.

Hysterectomy is not the operation you want to have when you

have abnormal bleeding. When cancer is suspected, these are risks you take to save your life.

> *I have a lump in my armpit. I've heard that this is the worst sign of breast cancer. Is that right?*

That lump may be a swollen lymph node, especially if you've been fighting an infection. It can be an infected hair follicle. Does it hurt? Often when you can touch an area and make it hurt, it's a sore muscle. In any case, the stress of wondering "Is it or isn't it?" really can make you sick. See your doctor.

> *Because I have so many of the risk factors for breast cancer, and my aunt died of it, should I get the new test that tells whether or not I carry the gene?*

The test you are referring to is a test for BRCA 1 and BRCA 2. Here's what this test is all about.

When three or more closely related individuals in a family have been diagnosed with breast cancer, it's likely that an inherited dominant genetic mutation is present. Mutations in the breast and ovarian cancer gene, BRCA 1, are believed responsible. An estimated 1 in 200 to 400 women in the United States have the BRCA 1 mutation and tend to develop breast cancer at a young age (under forty-five years). Environmental factors also play a key role, but studies indicate that women who carry the BRCA 1 gene have an 87 percent cumulative lifetime risk of developing breast or ovarian cancer. A second gene, BRCA 2, is also linked to early onset breast cancer but not to ovarian cancer.

For now, there are not many labs in the United States that have the expertise to do the tests for BRCA 1 and BRCA 2. Such testing is still in its infancy. And I'm not sure I'd recommend that you have it done in any case. First, the emotional fallout from being told you've tested positive can be devastating. And if you're positive, then what? If you don't currently have the disease, you can only take the same steps to reduce your risk that other women do. Some women want both breasts removed preventively.

One must also consider that people are sometimes denied health insurance on the grounds that they have a preexisting condition. Will an insurance company take a positive reading on this test as a preexisting condition? It's hard to know.

The key to fighting breast cancer is still detecting it at the earliest possible stage, which can best be done through mammograms, regular checkups, and monthly self-exams.

> *My doctor told me that I have a ten-week-size fibroid. What does that mean?*

Interns and residents are often trained in the O.R. by doing pelvic exams while patients are under anesthesia. Then the patient has an operation, and the intern gets to immediately see what he or she felt. As a doctor, you make a mental note about what certain conditions feel like. You do thousands of these exams in your training.

Pregnancies offer a standard for talking about the size of the uterus. *This feels like ten-week size. This feels like eight-week size.* So with fibroid tumors, doctors often describe the size of the uterus in terms of pregnancy. To describe a fibroid as being ten-week size means that the uterus has grown to the size that it would be in a ten-week pregnancy.

> *After going through saline-infusion sonohysterography, I was told I do need a D&C for therapy. Now what?*

Again, most women feel well enough the day after a D&C to go to work. And when a doctor removes a polyp, for example, he or she removes your problem. My suggestion, however, is that you make sure that the doctor is not going to do a D&C without hysteroscopy. If you are going to be subjected to the inconvenience and expense of a D&C, it shouldn't be blind scraping.

Hysteroscopy uses little instruments about the size of drinking straws that go inside the uterus and have fiberoptics attached to a light source. You put them on a little camera, and you can see the inside of the uterus on a TV screen. Using hysteroscopy, a doctor can see where exactly a polyp, for example, is and target it during the D&C.

> *What is the difference between a partial hysterectomy and a complete hysterectomy?*

I've heard doctors use these terms, but this is not medical terminology. When they say complete hysterectomy they mean the fallopian tubes and ovaries are removed as well as the uterus. When they say partial, they mean only the uterus. Hysterectomy truly only refers to removing the uterus.

*I've been told that I need a hysterectomy. Should I just say no and find another doctor?*

Not at all. But one thing is for sure: An informed patient can do a lot to distinguish between an appropriate hysterectomy and an inappropriate one.

What I want to stress here is that if you've been told you need a hysterectomy because of bleeding problems that don't go away, you want to know everything that can cause bleeding problems. You want to understand what can be done to diagnose them appropriately and rule out whether what you're experiencing is hormonal. The necessity for hysterectomy for bleeding is rare, as far as I'm concerned. Saline-infusion sonohysterography eliminates diagnostic guesswork beyond what a D&C can do. It's a test I highly recommend if you're told you need gynecological surgery.

*A friend told me that I don't need to worry about cancer of the cervix because I was a virgin until I was twenty-two. Is she right?*

No. It is true that one risk factor for cancer of the cervix is early sexual intercourse — in one's teens, for example — as well as multiple sex partners over one's lifetime. Other risk factors include having genital herpes, venereal warts, and smoking. There is also some evidence that women from lower socioeconomic groups have a greater incidence of cervical cancer, presumably secondary to the higher incidence of STDs (sexually transmitted diseases). Women who have sex with partners who are uncircumcised may also run a somewhat greater risk. But first intercourse at age twenty-two will not *protect* you.

# 8

# HOW TO GET THE MOST FROM MEDICAL SCIENCE — WHILE AVOIDING THE WORST

When I give lectures to groups of doctors across the country, I sometimes look out at the audience and wonder, "How many of these doctors still have the time to sit with a patient in her late thirties and forties in the consult room? How many still have the time to ask, 'How are you sleeping? Are you feeling a little off, not like your usual self? Having any problems with your memory?' "

These are important diagnostic questions for women in this age group, yet with managed care, doctors often aren't given enough time with patients to extract such subtle information. Soon the days of the doctor speaking with you in the consult room after every exam are going to be gone. For many that has already happened.

Chances are you have already had some experience with this. If you have health insurance, you are already or soon will be enrolled in some kind of managed care program. It may be a PPO — preferred provider program — where you pay less or even nothing at all to see a doctor who is part of your plan. Or you may be in an HMO — health maintenance organization — which limits which doctors you can see and why. Managed care, by definition, means that you and your doctor are now closely involved with a third party — your insurance company — in making choices about your health care, e.g., what specialists you can see, what tests will be covered, etc.

Almost gone are the days of hearing about a doctor from a friend, making an appointment, filling out an insurance form, and getting reimbursed. You may have to page through a book as large as your phone book when you hear of a doctor you want to see. You may find out he or she is not in your plan.

You may change jobs and find out your doctor is no longer covered under your new plan. You may feel that at a time when you have more questions, more health-related needs, your choices for help have never been more limited.

Although I choose *not* to participate in managed care, it is a reality that most doctors do. Managed care medicine in OB-GYN is a commitment to volume: Out of financial necessity, more people need to come through the door. Many physicians who have made a commitment to go through managed care in OB-GYN recognize the need for physician "extenders," such as nurse clinicians, physician assistants, videotape libraries in the waiting room, and quick put-through and turnaround. All of this affects what it feels like to be the patient. I'm sure that my grandfather, who died in 1948, would have been surprised if a friend had said to him, "Sam, someday when you're sick, you're going to have to get dressed and go to the doctor's office instead of having the doctor come to your house to see you." Sam would have said, "What, are you crazy? I am going to get out of my sickbed and go to a doctor?"

I believe the possibility exists that my daughter, Phoebe, who is a third grader, will never know the medical care that my patients still have access to. She will need to educate herself as much as possible about her health. For her, this will be commonplace and expected. For those of us in our forties and fifties, it's new and sometimes uncomfortable for our health care to be provided by people who are often strangers, who rely on us to tell our histories. As a patient, you may have little choice about participating in a managed care program if this is the insurance coverage you are offered through your employer. If you are content with your current doctor, but he or she isn't covered by your plan, you might attempt to maintain a point-of-service option so you can continue to see the doctor you are satisfied with out of network. It means you pay a higher deductible or copayment, but you can choose a doctor that doesn't participate in your plan. It's as close to old-fashioned major medical insurance as most people can obtain in today's arena, allowing you to retain as much choice as possible.

Managed care isn't going away. The debate over the benefits and drawbacks of managed care is beyond the scope of this book. But one thing is sure: Increasingly, it will be essential for *you* to be knowledgeable in order to be in control. If you position yourself as a selective consumer of health care, you can still get the best out of medical science — and avoid the worst.

Whatever your situation, you don't need to become an encyclopedia of modern medicine to get good health care. The information that follows in this chapter can help you make the most out of every gynecological appointment.

## How to Get the Best from Your Regular Appointment

I recommend you visit your OB-GYN twice a year. The most basic step in a thorough exam happens before you even make an appointment: Keep a good menstrual calendar. When a patient tells me she's "not that regular," it tells me very little. I can tell a lot from a good calendar. Record when you start to bleed and how many days you bleed. Add details about the lightness or heaviness of the flow if it has seemed unusual.

It's ideal if you can bring in the dates for the past year. If you are suffering from symptoms, you may want to chart those also. It can save you the time and money of a fishing expedition if you can show your doctor when symptoms such as sleeplessness, anxiety, or forgetfulness are occurring in relation to your menstrual cycle.

## Those Long Questionnaires — Should You Tell All?

The questionnaires you are often handed when you go to medical appointments are becoming longer and longer. Managed care has created a necessity for these longer forms, as the doctor tries to get as much information as possible before he or she sees you face-to-face.

The trouble is, these forms often seem invasive. There are women who are leery about putting things down in writing, especially when it comes to answering sensitive questions about sex or other aspects of personal history. It's one thing to answer in writing the question "Has anyone had heart disease in your immediate family?" and hand it back to a stranger; it's another to answer questions asking if you have had a sexually transmitted disease or unprotected sex with more than one partner.

The all-or-nothing yes/no answers on these questionnaires can be difficult. The patient reads, "Do you take any prescription drugs?" and the pen stops. She thinks, "Well, I felt jittery all week, and I took half of a Xanax out of the bottle my husband got when he hurt his back. So is this a yes or a no? Should I tell about my anxiety? Will the doctor think I'm bad because I'm taking someone else's drugs?"

Then there are the questions about personal habits. "Do you smoke?" You quit years ago, but you occasionally bum a couple of cigarettes when you go out for a drink after work. Is that a yes or a no? Do you need another lecture about smoking?

These forms ask for needed information, but no one is going to stop you from writing, "I'd like to discuss this in person" or drawing a big question mark on the form and waiting until you meet with your doctor to answer certain questions.

You are also free to ask why you're being asked certain questions. For example, "Doctor, your questionnaire asks about the use of recreational drugs. Can you explain how that might be related to changes in a woman's menstrual cycle?"

Just remember that when you are alone with your doctor, your health will benefit from complete disclosure. You can't get the best medical care if you withhold the information your doctor needs to help you.

Many women worry about being honest with their doctors. So much information is available about healthy habits and diets and lifestyles. Most of us fall short of perfection. If you don't know where your calcium is coming from because you haven't tasted milk in a decade, you haven't made time to get a mammogram, or you're fifteen pounds overweight, remember that you are the health-care consumer. You are not in your doctor's office to get a judgment about whether you have been good or bad, but how you can feel your best.

## What Should I Expect of a Good Exam?

When I meet a patient for the first time, I meet her in my office, clothed, not in the examining room. This is a courtesy women once took for granted. Now you may have to request it. If it bothers you to meet your doctor for the first time in the examining room, dressed in a gown, say so when you make the appointment.

In my opinion, the questionnaire most doctors give their patients, no matter how thorough, does not substitute for your doctor's asking if you have any concerns or having his or her own list of questions. I take my intake history by pen and paper, listening and watching during the interview. I learn a lot that questionnaires geared for scanning into a computer don't tell me. By the time I get to "Do you smoke?" I can tell you what the answer will be with 99 percent accuracy — even without smelling smoke on your clothes or seeing telltale signs on your teeth or fingernails.

Next, the nurse will generally check your blood pressure, height, and weight. You will usually be asked to provide a urine sample.

Most doctors begin their exam by examining your breasts. If you can time your appointment to the week after your period, when the tissue is least tender and lumpy, all the better. The worst time is the week before menstruation. Pressure on your breasts then can be uncomfortable.

I think it's important to do the breast exam with the patient both lying and sitting. I get a much different picture from each position. I can't tell you how often I have felt something in one position but not the other. Your doctor should spend at least a minute examining each breast, including the area around the nipples and armpits.

Where are most lumps found? In the upper, outer quarter of the breast, close to the armpit. If you don't do your own monthly exams, admit it. Women who don't do them complain that they have no idea what they're looking for or what they're supposed to feel. Or they're scared.

Doctors know that breast cancer is a frightening issue for women. Your doctor can tell you what to look for and show you how to do a good exam. I'm never shocked to hear a woman tell me that she doesn't examine herself because she doesn't really want to know. If you've skimped on your breast exams, don't allow your doctor to do so. Be reassured to know that the majority of lumps are benign fibrous tissue or fluid-filled cysts.

## What Is a Doctor Actually Looking For During a Pelvic Exam?

A thorough internal exam begins with your doctor examining the skin of the external vaginal area under a bright light. He or she is looking for any lumps, sores, bumps, or indications of an infection.

Next the doctor inserts the speculum into your vagina. After checking the vaginal walls and cervix for sores — such as white patches or ulcerations that look like canker sores — or a discharge that is unusual, a Pap smear is taken. Your doctor should collect cells from two places, the surface of the cervix and the inside of the canal that leads up into the uterus (called the endocervix).

Last comes the bimanual exam. The doctor inserts two gloved fingers into the vagina, places the other hand on your abdomen, and presses the pelvic organs. The doctor makes a mental image of what the pelvic findings are. Is this uterus tipped forward or backward? Is it normal in size? Is it normal in contour? Does each ovary or the region of each ovary feel like a normal size, or is something feeling enlarged? If it's enlarged, does it feel cystic or solid? Many doctors also include a fecal occult blood test as part of the exam.

## Is the Bimanual Exam Enough?

The bimanual pelvic exam at the gynecologist's office has consisted of the same thing for a hundred years: putting two fingers into the vagina and one hand on the lower abdomen in order to palpate the pelvic organs. Regardless of how good doctors are with their fingers and regardless of what they can tell about the size of the uterus, the location, and its general health from their experience and training, they can't see inside of it. And not all patients lend themselves to a meaningful palpatory examination. Some are overweight. Some do not relax enough.

My belief is that there are enormous benefits to using vaginal ultrasound as part of the routine exam. Any doctor with the right equipment and know-how can replace the subjective portion of the bimanual exam with an image in a matter of seconds. True, an image can't answer such questions as "Is this tender?" and "Is there normal mobility to these organs?" The bimanual exam is still important.

But ultrasound gives you more than just anatomic findings (size, shape, and configuration of the uterus and ovaries). For instance, if a woman is in the second half of her cycle, but on ultrasound examination the lining of the uterus is not compatible with ovulation and there is no evidence of ovulation in the ovary, then one can suspect anovulation.

I show each of my patients her "pictures" on ultrasound. Many women stare and nod without comprehension, because to the unpracticed eye the pictures look like clouds. In the future an understanding of these pictures can make a vital difference in the choices you make about your health. Don't be intimidated. You can absolutely understand what you see in those ultrasound pictures without too much struggle if you can be patient with a little medical jargon.

Let me walk you through the menstrual cycle as it appears on film. Realize that the ovary is a dynamic organ. At the beginning of the cycle, follicles, about a half dozen in each ovary, start to develop. These are small fluid-filled structures that appear cystic. The word *cyst* scares patients, but "cystic" really just means full of fluid, not the same as "tumor." These structures grow until about day nine of your cycle, when only one becomes dominant and starts to grow quickly until it reaches 2.5 cm. At that time, it should burst (ovulation) and release an egg. What you see on ultrasound is something thick and irregular. This is the corpus luteum. There may be some bleeding into the area where ovulation took place. The corpus luteum can expand due to the blood and take on a characteristic appearance known as the "corpus luteum cyst."

The estrogen your body produces causes the endometrial lining on ultrasound to go from being thin (4 to 5 mm) and single layered in appearance to being multilayered and halolike right before ovulation. The progesterone after ovulation causes this multilayered appearance to fill in, becoming somewhat peppered on the first two or three days and then very thick during the second half of the cycle. The lining that has built up is then shed (your period). At the end of the menses, when the endometrial cavity is empty, the sonogram will show a thin white line again. If there is still significant tissue after menstruation, one can discern this on ultrasound. This may be a polyp or hyperplasia. These are things that one could never detect with palpation alone.

By seeing into the lining of the uterus and correlating this with what is going on in the ovary, a doctor gets information about *function*, not just appearance. For instance, in the menopausal patient there will be no follicles discernible in the ovaries and there will be a thin white line for lack of significant tissue in the uterus. If a patient is perimenopausal and has no discernible follicles and a "pencil line" thin endometrial lining, this may mean low estrogen levels, not just anovulation. Patients on low-dose birth-control pills should have a predictable pattern of no follicles in the ovary and a very thin endometrial lining. (See the Appendix for examples of premenopausal and postmenopausal ultrasound images.)

Don't let the medical jargon confuse you. The point is, there should be correlation between what you see in the ovary and what you see in the lining of the uterus, since the lining of the uterus responds to the hormones or lack of hormones that the ovary is producing. Ultrasound exams are a way of providing women in transition with a more accurate means of diagnosing whether they are in fact in transition and assessing how that relates to any symptoms they may be experiencing. In addition, ultrasound can reveal unsuspected uterine tumors (fibroids) or ovarian enlargement whether functional (related to ovulation or lack thereof) or neoplastic (meaning new growth, whether benign or malignant).

I believe ultrasound enhancement of every pelvic exam will become a reality, although this may take more than a decade. Manufacturers are currently developing equipment that will be to current ultrasound machines what the laptop is to desktop computers, making such procedures available inexpensively to women everywhere for every exam.

## Do I Really Need That Test?

If you are in your late thirties or forties, there are a variety of tests your doctor may recommend.

## Mammograms

I recommend that you have your first mammogram by age forty unless there is family history of breast cancer on the maternal side, in which case you should have your first test at thirty-five. Your first mammogram provides a baseline against which any future changes can be measured and compared. The reason not to have a mammogram when you are younger is that younger women have very dense breast tissue, known as "parenchyma," and therefore these screenings are not very helpful.

How can you get the best out of a mammogram? Julie S. Mitnick, M.D., director of Murray Hill Radiology and Mammography in New York City and associate professor of clinical radiology at New York University Medical Center, gives this advice: "You should go to a mammography facility that is accredited by the American College of Radiology. They have standards in terms of the quality of the films that are produced. Your mammogram will be read by board certified radiologists." Approved facilities post a plaque. You can also call a facility and find out if it has such approvals before you make an appointment. Dr. Mitnick explains why this is important: "Much of whether something is seen on mammography or not depends on whether the films are done properly. The patient needs to be positioned properly. The processing of the films needs to be more than adequate. With subtle findings, it's very important that film is not overexposed or underexposed and that mammography is as good as it can be.

"Lumps usually occur at the upper margin of the breast, but they can occur anywhere. There are various ways that cancer can feel. Some cancers are very distinct, feel very hard, and are easy to discern on a clinical examination. Other cancers are very subtle. It may be a little thickening or a little modularity. Those are very difficult for the patient or her physician to pick up. Particularly it's hard if a patient has fibrocystic breast conditions, which is why mammography is so important. Some of the cancers we pick up are tiny, a single duct of the breast. These are cancers that you might not feel for years.

"The point of mammography is to detect cancer when it's smaller, when you can't feel it, when you have the best prognosis."

Perimenopause is a time when many women first become concerned about breast cancer. There are decisions to make about birth-control pills and, later, estrogen replacement therapy. The effect of estrogen on your breasts is usually of greatest concern. Suddenly a mammogram isn't just another test, like a Pap smear, but something more emotional, more frightening. At your relatively young age, with the media running stories about whether a mammogram will really do much for women in transitional years, you may think, "I'll just skip it." I hope you won't. You have every probability of gaining peace of mind.

To get the best out of your mammogram, don't use deodorant, powder, or lotion on the day of the exam. You don't want anything on your skin to interfere with a clear picture.

There are facilities that develop the film and give the results right there for those who cringe at the thought of getting results via voice mail or having to wait. Dr. Mitnik's staff speaks to each patient before she leaves. There is no reason why one has to wait for results other than choosing a facility that doesn't develop film immediately.

Any woman can also ask for her films. Even if you aren't experiencing any problems, you may want to keep them in your own medical file, stored flat, as a baseline against future exams and as part of your medical records.

If you are told that something is abnormal, don't be afraid to ask, "What exactly do you see?" and have the radiologist point it out on the film.

## When Mammograms Hurt

A good mammogram requires that your breasts be squeezed flat between two plates. Small-breasted women often complain that pushing all of the breast outward hurts. But the breast tissue must be pulled away from your chest to get the best picture. Women with dense breasts or who have engorged or tender breasts also may feel some discomfort. But proper positioning is everything with this test, and it's what highly trained technicians excel at.

If a mammogram hurts, it doesn't mean anything is wrong with your breasts. Think of the discomfort involved in getting the most tissue between the plates as insurance that you're getting a quality exam. Obviously, an experienced technician can make this whole procedure go faster, minimizing your discomfort.

## How to Do Your Own Breast Self-Exam

A mammogram isn't a substitute for monthly self-exams. How can you do a good self-exam? Wait until two or three days after your period. Stand before a mirror and look carefully at your breasts, noticing if there is anything that looks unusual. Squeeze your nipples. Is there a discharge? Is the nipple inverted in a way that's not normal for you? Do you notice any change in the shape of your breasts? Clasp your hands behind your head. Do you notice any dimpling or scaling of the skin on your breasts? Place your hands on your hips and look once more.

Lie on your back. Examine each breast with one hand, fingers flat, moving in a circular motion. Start at the outer edge and work your way in. Feel your underarm areas and the areas up to your collarbone. Do you feel anything unusual, a mass of tissue that feels fluid filled or moves under your fingers? Sit up and repeat the procedure.

## Cholesterol Measurements

It used to be that people were given a random cholesterol test, and if it was under 200 that was good. But we know now that there is good cholesterol — HDL — and bad cholesterol — LDL. It's better to get levels for both. My own last reading, for example, was 205, but that's because my HDL level (the good one) was so high. I like to see LDL less than 120 to 140 in my patients. (Total cholesterol = HDL + LDL + triglycerides ÷ 5. LDL is calculated, not measured.)

Besides estrogen, moderate exercise and moderate alcohol intake raise your good cholesterol. I remember the first time I heard that at a lecture. I turned to the doctor next to me and joked, "So the take-home message is jog to the liquor store." In any case, it's clear that you can do a fair amount about your cholesterol with diet and exercise.

Have a baseline test of your cholesterol by age forty. Then have it checked periodically. A person of forty-one, for example, with a wonderful cholesterol level does not have to be tested every year. A baseline at age forty is important to make sure you don't have some genetic or familial elevation, since genetics does play a role in this.

When I see a premenopausal woman who has an LDL of 165, for example, that's odd. It may not mean that she needs to take drugs, but it makes me take notice.

Cholesterol cannot be too low. No matter how low it is, it can always be lower. Some recent preliminary studies seem to indicate that the most important single factor is how high the HDL or good cholesterol is. Stay tuned.

## FSH Test

To understand why your doctor might recommend an FSH test, let's review the basics of hormonal happenings. To review, FSH stands for follicle stimulating hormone. On the first day of your period, when you start to bleed, estrogen and progesterone in your body are at their lowest levels. This signals the pituitary gland to begin producing FSH. The FSH stimulates the follicles to ripen and produce an egg. As the follicles ripen, they secrete estrogen. The estrogen is what causes the uterine lining to proliferate, which eventually becomes your period if fertilization does not take place.

Blood tests are often paradoxical in the following sense: I've known many patients who have estradiol levels that are not in a menopausal range (in other words, they are still making estrogen), but their FSH levels have started to rise. (FSH in premenopause is less than 30.) According to the laboratories' norms, they are menopausal. It is paradoxical because although the patient's estrogen level is premenopausal, the patient's FSH is postmenopausal. This is typical of transition.

## Pap Test — New Developments Mean Greater Health

You probably had your first Pap test in your twenties. Sometimes women think that since this test is so commonplace, such a regular part of their exams, it's okay to skip it — or not go in for your annual exam at all.

The highest rate of incidence of cervical cancer is between the ages of thirty-five and fifty-five. With regular Pap tests, in which cervical cells are examined for cancerous changes, you can eliminate your chances of developing cervical cancer. This is because before cancer develops, there is a precancerous stage that produces cellular changes in the cervix. By taking a sample of cells from the cervix annually and examining them under a microscope, doctors can identify abnormalities and treat them before they develop into cancer since these cells are slow growing.

There have been some changes and advances in Pap tests over the last decade. While the most common instrument used to collect the sample cells is still the cotton swab, some doctors also use two new instruments. One resembles a small wooden spatula and the other a tiny brush. The importance of collecting cells from two areas of the cervix has also been underscored and is now a regular practice.

The vocabulary used in disseminating Pap smear results has also changed. Formerly, results were divided into five classes. Class I meant normal; class II was atypical; classes III and IV were different levels of dysplasia, which is the abnormal precancer change of the cervix; and class V was a Pap smear that suggested actual cancer.

If a Pap test does not come back from the lab classified as normal, it can carry one of the following results:

1) ASCUS (atypical squamous cells of undetermined significance). Fifty to sixty percent of abnormal Pap results are ASCUS. ASCUS shouldn't be confused with abnormal or cancerous. This means there are some cells the doctor sees on the slide that aren't typical. It may be that the nucleus of a cell is irregular or enlarged, or that the cytoplasm stains in an unusual fashion (at the lab, an automated wheel dunks Paps into a series of staining solutions that allow the technician to read them). This can be due to a vaginal infection that requires antibiotics or some other mild treatment. The doctor doesn't feel the cells are precancerous — if she did she would label them that way — but she is unwilling to label them as a normal Pap smear.

If your result comes back ASCUS, some doctors recommend repeating the test after an interval of six weeks to two or three months. If there are two ASCUS results in a row, most clinicians recommend colposcopy. Be aware, however, that ASCUS readings are becoming more common: Don't panic. In truth, the growth in the number of ASCUS results may have to do with the fact that labs feel the need for protection against lawsuits in a litigious society.

Colposcopy is the use of low-powered magnification to view the cervix. It allows for an eight- to forty-fold magnification of the cervix, a way for a doctor to see inflammation, infection, or polyps. The apparatus looks like little binoculars. Weak acetic acid is also used during the procedure. Most abnormal lesions of the cervix are known as "aceto white," meaning they will turn white with the application of 3 to 5 percent acetic acid. In addition, abnormal lesions of the cervix do not take up a strong iodine, also known as Lugol's iodine. That is also used to determine lesions that may be suspicious. If at the time of colposcopy the doctor notices aceto white lesions, these are biopsied at the same time. In addition, the doctor may scrape up the endocervical canal, where he or she can't see, and send this tissue to the lab to be sure there is no disease up in the canal.

2) Low-grade SIL and high-grade SIL. These correspond to the old class III and IV categorizations. SIL stands for "squamous intraepithelial lesions." This means that the cervical cells show some abnormality. "Low-grade" and "high-grade" refer to the degree of abnormality.

To fully understand this, one needs to understand the word "squamous." The exocervix (the bump you can feel if you insert a finger deep into your vagina) and the vagina are lined with squamous tissues. This tissue is somewhat protective, like the inside of your cheek. The cervix is constantly laying down new squamous tissue to repair and heal itself. The endocervix (the portion of the cervical canal that leads up into the actual uterine cavity) is lined with tall cells called "columnar epithelium." They are responsible for making the cervical mucus that brings the sperm to meet the egg. Virtually all precancerous changes of the cervix arise at the junction of the squamous and columnar epithelium. Still, keep in mind that conditions like vaginitis or yeast infections can cause abnormal readings; SIL doesn't mean cancer.

3) Suspicious for malignant cells. This means changes in the cells that suggest cancer.

One point needs to be stressed: If you have an abnormal Pap smear (not ASCUS, which is atypical and can be repeated), don't bother repeating the test. If a repeat Pap smear fails to show the abnormal cells seen on the initial one, why would you believe that any more than the original? The cells do not fall out of the sky onto your slide. An abnormal (not atypical) Pap smear should be followed by a colposcopy, not a repeat smear.

Keep in mind that a Pap smear result isn't absolutely a diagnosis. There have been studies where ten doctors looked at the same slide, and some labeled it low-grade SIL, others high-grade SIL. There is still a lot of subjectivity here. Generally, a technician will read the slide first. If he or she deems it abnormal, it will be screened again by a doctor.

Think of colposcopy as a more in-depth study of the cervix. A cone biopsy may be performed if the colposcopy reveals cancerous tissue or is inconclusive. This means that a piece of your cervix in the shape of a cone is removed, using a laser or scalpel, while you are under anesthesia. If these cells are abnormal, treatment can include destroying the abnormal cells by freezing them; laser surgery, which uses a laser beam to destroy the cells; or electrocoagulation, which uses heat to destroy the cells.

Because Pap smears aren't 100 percent reliable, every woman can benefit by preparing for them in a way that will at least eliminate some of the known problems that throw off results. First, schedule your appointment for one week after the end of your period. Don't douche or use talc in the vaginal area, and avoid any vaginal medication, including lubricants and contraceptive creams, for twenty-four hours before your exam. It is best not to have sexual intercourse the night before the exam.

Realize that you can be called back to retake a Pap test just because it is unreadable. There may have been blood present, or you may have had a gynecological infection. Sometimes cells are collected from the wrong part of the cervix.

Also, if you have a history of genital warts, make sure your doctor knows this. Genital warts are caused by the human papilloma virus (HPV), which can cause changes in cells that show up in your Pap test.

It's unfortunate that many women think a Pap smear is something they can skip after having their children. It is especially important if you are having sex with multiple partners or unprotected sex, or if you've had a sexually transmitted disease. Again, if we can catch cervical changes at the precancerous stage, the tissue can be removed without major surgery.

## Questions Women Ask

*I've heard so many horror stories lately about false negatives on Pap tests. Can I really trust my results?*

Some of these false negatives were due to technicians (cytotechnologists, or cytotechs) reading too many slides in one day, or doctors collecting too few cells or only sampling one part of the cervix.

Ask your doctor if he or she intends to sample more than one area of the cervix when you go in for your Pap. You can also inquire about the lab your doctor uses. There are now laws in all states that limit the number of slides a cytotech can examine to 100 a day. You can ask your doctor how many slides are screened per day at the lab where your cells are examined.

*I don't want to spend money for unnecessary tests. What should I ask my doctor when she tells me I should have certain tests done?*

Ideally you want a physician who knows what to ask you or tell you. Still, here are good, reasonable questions to ask:

1) Why do you recommend that I take this test? What are you looking for? Why do you think I need this test to get this information?

2) How will I find out the results? By phone? Mail?

3) If the test is negative, does it mean I definitely don't have the condition or that it just isn't showing up in this test? Where will we go from there?

4) How often will I need this test?

5) How much does this test cost? Will my insurance cover it? Will your office call to verify coverage, or do I call?

6) Will I feel well enough to drive home by myself after the test?

# 9

# SEX, SEXUALITY, AND FERTILITY

Alicia wasn't really counting, but she was sure she and Brad hadn't had sex for two months. Maybe three.

She held a folder full of airline tickets and travel vouchers in her hand and thought about seven nights in Saint Thomas. Hot afternoons, no kids, no interruptions, no TV. A time to reconnect sexually.

What happened? "We made love that first afternoon and then again the next morning. Seven days flew by. We played tennis, we swam, we had wonderful meals. We never got around to sex again. I thought that with no interruptions, we'd have sex three times a day. It wasn't that he lost interest. Both of us did. What happened?"

There are afternoons when Eileen disappears into her bedroom, lies down on the bed, and thinks about sex with Ryan. The other night at dinner, when their hands touched accidentally, she felt eighteen again. How long had it been since she wanted someone badly?

Trouble is, Ryan is her neighbor's new boyfriend. It's a crazy adolescent crush, but it's entering into her thoughts dozens of times a day. She'd never actually *do* anything about what she feels, but what scares her is that these fantasies are so compelling.

She truly loves her husband. The sex they have doesn't rock the world, but she enjoys it, and he says he does too. Still, Ryan is in her head. She can't get him out. "I keep dreaming about great sex — the kind you have when you first fall in love, when you want somebody so much it almost hurts. It depresses me to think that I'm never going to feel that again."

Claire found herself heavily involved in relationships with two men when she was in her early twenties. Brian was moody, cerebral, exciting in a dark, unpredictable way. Karl was her steady, affectionate lover, a man who adored children, worked hard for good money, and didn't mind doing the dishes. Karl made her feel special. Brian made her feel like she was never good enough.

"Sex with Brian was always exciting, but we never had sensitive sex like I had with Karl. I started to cry in the middle of it once, and Brian got out of bed and went to get himself a beer. Karl would never have done that. I knew that I would be crazy to let Karl's kind of love go."

She married Karl. Their life together was good. "We adore our kids. We connect in so many ways. But our sex life turned into nothing. It's like we're roommates.

"I catch him looking at me sometimes, when he doesn't think I'm watching. He looks hurt, confused, expectant. It's hard to face the fact that he's probably disappointed too. He wants something from me I just can't give him right now. I wonder if I made the wrong choice. Lately I don't feel sexual at all."

Kevin and Lisa are soul mates. They work together. They've remodeled two homes together. At forty-five, they have no children, but their two Labradors have the run of their home. They are busy building their business, entertaining their friends. They view themselves as child-free rather than childless.

Lately, though, Lisa has begun to worry about the lack of sex in their relationship. "We can go two months and not have it, then have it for a week or two, and then another dry spell. He isn't complaining. I'm not complaining. But you read stuff, you know? Two times a week is the norm, they say. Are we abnormal? Are we headed for affairs and some midlife crisis? This might sound strange, but what bothers me about the lack of sex is that it doesn't bother me."

## Is It Hormonal?

Many women tell me there has been no change in their sex drive during transition or after it. There are also women who tell me that sex is better than ever. Research on whether perimenopause contributes to a lack of sexual desire is in its infant stages. One study, *A Mid-life Women's Health Survey*, conducted through Penn State University, found that of their 505 participants ages thirty-five to fifty-five, only 25 percent said they were less interested in sex now than in their younger years.

Many women tell me that they are more comfortable about sex, more at ease after the embarrassment of earlier years. In addition, many say they feel more deserving of a good sex life as they get past their thirties.

But there are women who say they could take most sex or leave it. They wonder if a diminished yearning for the partner they used to feel crazy about is hormonal.

When a patient tells me she rarely feels sexual when she wants to, the first thing I want to rule out is medical causes. This is another of those perimenopausal symptoms that may not be all in your head.

## Is a Prescription or Over-the-Counter Drug Secretly Sapping Your Desire?

Researchers say that 50 to 75 percent of sexual problems have a physical rather than psychological cause. Often that cause is medication. Sexual side effects of medication are more common than we think, and they are the least reported. Many people are shy about mentioning a lack of sexual desire or inhibited sexual performance to their doctors, so the correlation isn't always made.

Here are some of the most common drugs that have been cited by women as affecting their sex drive:

1) Antihistamines. The same cold medicine or allergy pill that dries up your runny nose can make you feel dry everywhere. Dry vaginal membranes make sex uncomfortable.

When you don't lubricate easily, you may think you're not turned on by your partner. But are your eyes dry? Do you have a dry cough, a thirst nothing quenches? Look to your antihistamine when sexual lubrication doesn't happen. Dryness is a side effect of antihistamines; it doesn't mean you're falling out of love.

It's true that dryness in the vagina is often caused by lack of estrogen, the precursor to menopause. But women who have sufficient estrogen may think they are menopausal because their vaginas are dry when in reality the dryness could be related to other reasons. When a woman's body stops making estrogen, there will be some drying of the vagina, but this is not an overnight occurrence; it happens over time.

2) Antidepressants. Seventeen percent of people taking Prozac report the loss of sexual desire. The other antidepressants in the same class — Zoloft, Paxil, Serzone — can have the same effect. There are also people on these antidepressants who are so relieved to feel like themselves once again that they feel sexual for the first time in years. But as many as 30 percent of women, depending on which study you read, experience an inhibition of orgasm when on these particular drugs. As one woman put it, "I'd get to the brink and then, all of a sudden, nothing. It was so frustrating."

Sometimes changing to a different antidepressant helps. Some people report success taking a "weekend off" from the drug, although you should consult your doctor before changing dosages or regimens.

Being understanding with yourself is key. Depressed and despondent, chances are you weren't in the mood either. You aren't going to be on the medication forever, and helping your partner understand this potential side effect of your medication can do much toward diminishing a sense of failure in either of you.

3) Antibiotics. When you're taking an antibiotic because you feel ill, the illness itself can diminish sexual desire. There's nothing in an antibiotic that has been linked to sexual problems. But in many women, antibiotics clear up the infection only to cause an overgrowth of vaginal yeast.

Although it is called a yeast infection, it's not truly an infection. By killing some of the normal bacteria in the vagina, the antibiotic allows yeast forms that live there to multiply, and you end up with an itching or burning sensation.

The last thing a woman with such a yeast "infection" wants to think about is sex, because more often than not it hurts. Over-the-counter remedies can diminish symptoms in as little as three days.

The medications put the bacteria and yeast in the vagina back into balance, although they don't cure anything.

The difference between curing and putting the vagina back into balance is an important distinction to understand. Because we use the word *infection* with yeast, women think they have "caught" it. When they take medication and the itching goes away, they think the yeast is gone. But yeast is a normal inhabitant of 85 percent of women's vaginas. When it gets out of balance with other bacterial organisms, it can cause irritation, itch, and cottage cheese–like discharge. The medications put things back into balance in that they help get rid of the overgrowth of yeast. They do not eliminate it from the vagina; it is a normal inhabitant, and it will still live there.

4) Birth-control pills. Whether birth-control pills enhance or inhibit sex drive is still a subject of debate. Knowing you can't get pregnant when you don't want to can be a plus for your sex drive. But some women report a diminished desire for sex when they begin taking the Pill, or when they are no longer bleeding.

There are researchers who have concluded that the strong surge in hormones during ovulation creates an enhanced sexual desire — nature's way of continuing the species. Since the Pill stops ovulation, the spike in hormones doesn't happen.

If you are experiencing side effects of the Pill, such as bloating, you are understandably less in the mood. Sometimes taking a different pill or a different dosage diminishes side effects.

5) Alcohol. A glass of wine with dinner, when this is nothing new for you, can heighten desire, make you feel relaxed. Three or four, and you're experiencing what alcohol truly is: a major depressant.

Here is what one woman, who was at the brink of success in her sales career and at the depths of failure in her marriage, told me: "There were drinks after a hard day at work, drinks during a business meeting, a glass of wine while romancing a new client; I put dinner together and got the kids in bed, and I was exhausted. All that alcohol, so relaxing during the day, added up to feeling too tired for anything remotely tied to sex at bedtime. I just wanted to lie there, floating, uncaring, and alone."

Anyone who drinks regularly and is experiencing a loss of sexual desire should take stock of how much she is drinking and whether it's the culprit for a lack of libido. As this woman put it, "When I quit all the business drinking, all of my senses were heightened. I felt less tired, more alive, more interested in sex. I save the wine for special occasions now. I'm learning to control that anxious, tired feeling in other ways."

6) Other drugs — notably those for hypertension or to treat ulcers — can also contribute to a lowered sex drive.

If you find that a medication is causing a lack of sexual desire, ask yourself: What physical problems am I trying to ameliorate with this drug? Is it working? What are my priorities? Is it worth it to feel less sexual arousal to rid myself of other symptoms? Do I have a choice?

## Unopposed Estrogen and Sex

You feel cranky. Your breasts are so tender you can't wear your bra. You feel fat from retaining water. You're waiting for your period, because once it comes you feel better. But nothing happens. You go over your calendar. You wonder if you've gotten your dates mixed up. Forty days after your last period, this one finally arrives. You pass a huge clot and wonder if you were pregnant. Not exactly the portrait of a woman yearning for sex.

There is no data that tie a perimenopausal woman's hormonal fluctuations to a lack of sex drive. Still, if you're having all of the symptoms of a period that doesn't come, it is little wonder that sex is the last thing on your mind. I recommend that you see your doctor to find out what steps you can take to restore your equilibrium first, before you decide that your sex drive or your partner is the culprit.

## When Sex Hurts

Sex is uncomfortable for some women in transition. The most common complaint is that lubrication takes longer than it used to. This can occur as early as age thirty-five or so.

This is one of the physical changes of age, not unlike drier skin. You may be as turned on as ever by your partner, but lubrication isn't what it used to be. Trouble comes when you don't attribute this change to hormonal fluctuations and blame it on difficulty becoming aroused by your partner. It is normal during midlife to experience decreased vaginal secretions, even when you are otherwise aroused. In a poll conducted by *The Journal of Sex and Marital Therapy*, 40 percent of respondents said that lack of vaginal lubrication was a main factor inhibiting orgasm.

Don't put yourself through episodes of dry, painful sex. You may begin to associate sex with discomfort. My patients tell me that Astroglide is the best lubricant — although some people have success with K-Y jelly, Replens, or other brands. The good news is that there is no evidence that a woman's age affects her capacity to have an orgasm. There have even been studies that claim a woman's capacity to climax increases with age.

## Testosterone — Passion Pill?

Testosterone is the hormone that puts hair on a man's chest, bigger muscles in his arms, and energy into his sex drive. Why are women suddenly asking their doctors for it?

Women also make small amounts of testosterone, about one-twentieth of what men make. When menopause begins, some women (some researchers say as many as 50 percent) stop producing testosterone, while others keep producing it. No one knows why. Testosterone became big news when several studies found that postmenopausal women taking synthetic testosterone had higher levels of sexual desire, arousal, and fantasy, and made love more often than those taking a placebo.

Some women who have their ovaries removed experience a very noticeable drop in their sex drive, which is lessened when they're given testosterone. Today, prescriptions for Estratest, an estrogen/methyltestosterone combination pill, are being filled at the rate of over two million a year in the U.S.A.

So where does this leave you? First, the key word here is *menopause*, which is when testosterone production may well dip. If you're not there yet, and your ovaries are still producing hormones, there's a good chance that you are producing the testosterone you need as well. Research on testosterone and women is in its infancy, and even though I may prescribe it, I can tell women little about long-term effects. I can warn them, however, that testosterone has a tendency to lower HDL, the good cholesterol levels, when taken in pill form, so this needs to be monitored. I can also tell you that 50 percent of the women taking it see no change in libido, according to research. Still, a fifty-fifty chance may seem large if a low sex drive is interfering with the quality of your life.

It would be wonderful if we could test you and tell you whether your testosterone levels were low. Unfortunately, today's tests are not very accurate for the low levels of testosterone women have in their bodies. There is generally no way to compare them with what you used to have, since a test for testosterone is not something one is naturally given in one's thirties.

When a woman tells me she has absolutely no interest in sex, I ask if this was also true a decade ago. If she tells me, "To be honest, sex was never such a big deal," testosterone is not going to be the answer, even in the most hopeful patient, because she always had the hormone in her body and it didn't seem to do the job. When a woman can pinpoint that her lack of interest in sex coincided with menopause, I think of supplementary testosterone as one possible remedy.

Doctors prescribe testosterone in a pill, usually Estratest, which combines estrogen and methyltestosterone. Shots of testosterone can also be administered, but they seem to wear off in a few days. There are implants a doctor can place under your skin, and patches are now undergoing clinical trials. Supplementary testosterone is like estrogen therapy; if you want the maximum benefit, you need to keep taking it.

You may want to keep your eye on research coming out on testosterone and discuss it with your doctor. But at your age — isn't it nice to be too young for something? — and biological stage, I can't recommend that you take more of something you already have enough of.

## If It Isn't My Health, How Come I'm Not Interested in Sex?

Your sex drive isn't solely dependent on your hormones. Your expectations, perceptions, and emotions play a big part.

Are you rushed, overworked, and constantly tired? This can be the road to sexual turnoff — and it is the lifestyle of many women today. One patient told me she looks forward to an evening alone in bed with her laptop more than with her husband. "Sex has no purpose — it's an hour taken away from the things I need to do. I resent it, because he always seems to wander in demanding sex when I'm in the middle of a spreadsheet. An hour at the gym has a purpose — I can burn off calories on the StairMaster and really accomplish something. Helping my kid with homework — well, that's a priority these days. Sex I could take or leave."

While your feelings may not be that extreme, you are not alone if you are so busy these days that the thought of stopping your activities to have sex seems impossible, because you don't have time to waste. One patient told me that since her second child was born, her sexual activities have shifted from late night to early morning. "I tell him, if you want me, you better take me now. By nine o'clock tonight there's going to be nothing left."

If you're balancing family and career, chances are you often feel overwhelmed. Chicago-based psychotherapist Susan Piser, M.A., who has counseled couples for more than two decades, believes that for many partners, exhaustion is the core lovemaking problem. "Most women I talk to who have children are really tired, physically tired. At the end of the day they do not have an awful lot of time left over for *themselves*. That's first and foremost. They don't feel terribly feminine; they don't feel terribly womanly. There's a big shift in what's a priority. Maybe going to the kid's soccer game *is* more of a priority than making love. Maybe getting a balanced meal on the table *is* more of a priority. There are women who don't have children but are focused on their careers and have hit a crucial point after years of waiting for it to happen. That too can take precedence."

According to Piser, it's natural rather than unhealthy for sex to go on the back burner sometimes. When she counsels couples who complain of the loss of sexual desire, she encourages them to look at the total picture of what's going on in their lives. "There's generally a lot going on psychologically in the decade before menopause. Women are constantly reassessing everything, their careers, their marriages, their relationships with their parents, their children."

## A Good Sex Life Isn't All or Nothing

Many women are confused by magazine surveys reporting that "average" married couples have sex twice a week (or some other number, depending on which magazine you're reading). Like many of my patients, you may think, "Really? Not me. What's wrong with my marriage?"

But Piser says, "I don't know that there's any way you can quantify what the average married couple is doing or what the average is. I know people who go through three or four months without having any sex at all, people who have it sporadically, people who don't have it for a while and then have it a lot for a while. My sense is there is less sex going on than most people would like to acknowledge. What is normal is what's normal for you and your mate."

Less interest in sex doesn't necessarily mean the relationship is in trouble, despite an avalanche of magazine articles that would have you believe otherwise. "If a woman tells me that she used to feel very passionate about her husband, but lately she has little interest in sex, even though she's in love and otherwise happy, I'm apt to say, 'It's not the end of the world. You're feeling other stuff that is as significant,' " says Piser.

Piser believes that it's more difficult than most people realize to have a profound emotional connection and a profound physical connection simultaneously. "If you are very emotionally connected to someone, sometimes you need some distance. Pulling away sexually creates that distance. If you are really hooked into someone emotionally, to be hooked in physically at the same time can be difficult. It makes people feel too vulnerable.

"If you are feeling strongly connected physically, then you may not feel that connected emotionally. In good marriages it can go back and forth between the two. But there are a lot of people who opt for one or the other. They opt for a good, solid emotional connection and feel, 'It's okay; we have sex some of the time.' But to feel very intimate and very vulnerable with someone on a bunch of different levels simultaneously is much too scary for a lot of people."

What about the couple who went on vacation imagining that

they'd have sex three times a day and then only had it twice? What went wrong?

According to Piser, maybe nothing. "The fantasy was that this vacation was going to be way more sexual — not necessarily way more meaningful — than they thought. They got there and they connected physically. My hunch would be if it didn't happen again and no one is complaining, well, there are many more ways couples can relate and connect. If it's a good vacation, and they are having a great time, then sex might just not seem that important."

Piser has this advice for women at this stage of life: "Accept that sex isn't going to be amazing every time — and you aren't going to want it every minute. You don't have to accept the end of passion entirely. There's all kinds of passion. If you're with a partner you want to be with, sex can evolve in a bunch of different ways. You will go through periods where you are not that interested. You don't feel swept away when he walks in the door, but this doesn't mean there isn't a solid sexual relationship. If you have sex that is fun, feels good, and is emotionally connected, then you're on solid ground."

## When One of You Wants More

Sexual drive varies greatly from couple to couple. If neither you nor your mate is complaining about sex, then there is probably no reason to believe that your marriage or partnership isn't viable, even if you're having little sex. The trouble is, in many relationships someone is complaining. In fact, researchers find that in most couples there is one person who believes he or she is more interested in sex and more rejected than the other.

Mitch Meyerson, L.C.S.W., who has run relationship effectiveness groups in the Midwest for the past fifteen years and is the coauthor of *When Is Enough, Enough?*, believes sex isn't always the real issue. "Often sexual problems in couples are really emotional power plays," he says. "A couple may come in, and the man will say, 'She never wants to have sex. She's never interested.' But when I watch them relate to each other, something else emerges. He makes a lot of statements about where she falls short, how she isn't enough. He tries to control her without even realizing that he is doing it.

"It's my hunch that this woman withholds sex as an unconscious way of saying, 'I'm not enough? Well, I'll show you that you're not enough.' In the course of therapy, as she learns to speak up and talk about these issues, sex is no longer the battleground."

While the stereotype today is *He wants more; she wants less*, it can work both ways. It can even meet an unconscious need in the relationship. Piser says, "I can't tell you how many couples I've seen where the complaint is 'I'm not having enough sex,' and then when you look more carefully at it, the couple has an investment in seeing one partner as the rejecting one.

"For example, a woman may be unconsciously invested in seeing her partner as powerful. So if the partner is holding out on her, that maintains that image. Or he is invested in seeing her as unattainable, or powerful in a more maternal way. The unconscious motivation tends to be more complicated than what is on the surface. I find that people who are attracted to one another can tolerate the same level of distance or closeness. Usually, if they're talking quantity, it's pretty okay with both of them the way they're handling it, at least in viable marriages, even if someone is complaining."

How can one assess whether unconscious power plays are causing a lack of sexual interest? Piser asks partners how they approach each other when they want sex. "Most couples, if they really want to seduce one another, know how to do it. If you know your wife doesn't like to be grabbed and you come up in the kitchen and grab her, unconsciously you know you are going to push her away.

"Since it's not conscious, you will feel, 'Why is she rejecting me?' but you have to look at the behavior. Chances are, unconsciously you don't want it any more than she does."

Dampened sexual desire can also be caused by fear, anxiety, and insecurity. The antidote? Communication. Letting go of secret resentments, sharing the stress you feel, having private time together, letting your partner know what you're feeling, can help you connect again if you've drifted apart.

## When Your Body Gets in the Way

Julie, forty-two, had the kind of metabolism at thirty that seemed to burn up everything she ate. Not so at forty. For the first time in her life she is taking exercise and diet seriously, but it is a slow process.

She says this about sex with her partner: "Sometimes he pulls me over on top of him. He thinks this should excite me. Do you know what a woman my age looks like on top? I can't get this weight off, and my stomach just hangs there. It makes me sick. I want it over quickly. Even on 'thin days' I want the lights out."

Feeling physically self-conscious is a downer when it comes to sex, for men and women. You don't want the lights on; you don't want him to see you naked. You definitely don't want to experiment with different, more revealing positions. Even with the simplest sex, you can't relax.

Subtle physical changes — weight gain and/or changes in shape from childbearing or surgery — can play a role in diminished sexual desire. The idea that your body may turn someone off can make you feel that sex isn't worth the added vulnerability and anxiety. Many women are worried that their bodies don't measure up to an impossible ideal. Instead of focusing on intimacy, they fix their attention on the way they look to their partners.

What can you do? If your body's appearance is preventing you from enjoying sex, you have two options. You can work psychologically to learn to accept yourself as you are and become more comfortable with the body you have. Or you can work physically to make your body the best it can be so you feel better about it. I'm not talking about perfection, but a body that's as fit and healthy as you can make it.

There's a fine line between these two. I have patients who are physically fit, at their most desirable weight, and are still obsessed with cellulite, tiny imperfections, problem areas no one would notice were they not pointing them out. I've also had patients who are comfortable with their bodies in spite of vast changes from multiple children, weight gain, scars, etc. And there are women I've met who have terrible body images in their own minds, yet are having great sex lives.

What matters is what you're feeling about yourself and how that affects your sex life. How you feel about your body can have vast ramifications for your sexuality. Are you being realistic? Ask yourself these questions:

- Have you always criticized your body, even when the trouble spots that glare at you today didn't exist?

    For example, one woman showed me a picture of herself at twenty-two. She stood in shorts and a halter top on a sailboat, her long blond hair blowing in the wind. She didn't have an ounce of body fat that I could see. Her comment? "I thought I was fat in those days. I was obsessed with my thighs."

    This woman is toned and fit, and at forty-five has a face that is only beginning to show some of the stresses of age. She realizes that her preoccupation with her appearance has always limited her. It covers a deeper anxiety about the lack of control she has often felt in her life. A small salad without dressing means she's in control. A hot fudge sundae means she's out of control. Her life has become more or less a fight for control, and she deprives herself of any fun — and sex is part of that — when she feels she's let go of control.

    Women painfully preoccupied with physical defects can become more concerned about keeping their stomachs flat during sex than enjoying the experience. With a new mind-set, they can realize that they are much more than their bodies, that they are desirable simply for who they are.

- Have you become uncomfortable with your body recently, as a result of childbearing or a midlife weight gain or surgery?

    Give yourself time to adapt. Give your body time to get back into its natural rhythms. Be patient with yourself.

- Have other people told you more than once that you look fine, that you're unrealistic?

    "I wish my wife would lose weight," a patient's husband recently told me. "I don't need her to, but she's so miserable that she talks about it all of the time. I love having a family. I can see that her body has changed since she had our children, but it doesn't bother me the way it bothers her. I'd take my wife any day over some skinny twenty-five-year-old, but she doesn't believe that."

Do men notice the extra ten pounds, the stretch marks, the whatever else? Yes, some of them do. And don't you notice their love handles, receding hairlines, etc.?

When I talk to the husbands and partners of my patients, I hear over and over again that they don't find the aging body's flaws a big problem. What's more undesirable is the constant obsession and nit-picking:

"She asks how she looks in a dress. I say, 'Fine.'"

"She says, 'What do you mean *fine?* Does it look tight?'"

"I say, 'No, you look good.'"

"She says, 'What do you mean *good?*'"

"I say, 'You look okay, and we're going to be late, so can we just go?' But the truth is, now I'm getting pissed. It isn't what she wants to hear.

"Why is this always an issue? Let her go on a diet and stick to it if she doesn't like her stomach. This dialogue goes on for a half hour, or we end up in a major fight. Whatever I say, it's never enough."

When you can't take in any reassurance, when the way you look affects every aspect of your happiness, it's time to give yourself a much-needed break.

Everyone in this culture — man or woman — is affected by TV, movies, magazines. You are looking at air-brushed bodies almost every time you see a photo in a magazine. You need to accept that there are people who are a decade or more younger than you, who are childless, or have three hours a day to exercise with personal trainers because their bodies are their livelihoods.

Your life may be very different. You may not have three hours a day to sculpt your body because your body is not your priority. Those three hours may go into bathing your children, working at your computer, getting a balanced meal on the table, straightening out your house, meeting with new clients. Perfect is not the goal. Health is the goal. Make your priority getting some balance in your life so that you can make your body the healthiest and most toned that is reasonable for you.

## The Biological Clock

Women in their late thirties or forties who are not yet married often ask about the "biological clock." I truly believe this: First you should find a soul mate. Once you're a couple, couples sometimes decide to become families. When the two of you do, you look for whatever options are available, whether it's becoming pregnant naturally or moving on to high-tech reproductive technologies or adoption.

There is much in medical science to help you have a family. I would caution any woman against putting the cart before the horse — going out and having a baby, especially without a committed partner, just because statistics say she has only a few more years in which she can become pregnant.

A woman's chance of conceiving naturally within a year over the age of forty is 25 to 30 percent. Still, midlife motherhood is definitely on the rise. I have had patients in their late thirties and early forties who conceived the first time they had unprotected sex, merely by carefully charting their menstrual cycles and having sex on the appropriate days. However, it's estimated that 75 percent of women over forty will need some help from technology to conceive.

What makes it so difficult to have a baby during perimenopause? First and foremost, you may not ovulate every month, giving you fewer chances to become pregnant. Next, women simply have fewer and older, less viable eggs. A woman is born with more than a million eggs, but by the time of perimenopause it's estimated that she has about ten thousand left. Less viable eggs are those that are harder for sperm to penetrate.

Some women have scar tissue that comes from the ovary having to repair itself after each ovulatory cycle. The more difficult a time the egg has navigating through this scar tissue to the place where it can be released, the more difficult conception becomes. Scarring can also come from pelvic inflammatory disease, caused by sexually transmitted diseases such as chlamydia. If it goes untreated for long, it can cause enough scarring to block the fallopian tubes or damage the ovaries. The fallopian tubes, which link the ovaries to the uterus, must be unobstructed for pregnancy to occur.

The cervix can also cause problems. If it is scarred from previous childbirths or narrowed for any reason, it can block the sperm from reaching the egg. In rare cases, a woman's cervical mucosa contains substances that immobilize sperm.

Many women of perimenopausal age have had gynecological surgery. If you've had a fibroid or some other benign growth removed, there may be scar tissue as a result.

Your body is probably still making estrogen in perimenopause — and progesterone when you ovulate. But how high are those levels? It's not uncommon for women to find that they don't secrete enough progesterone to prepare the endometrium for the fertilized egg. The egg can't embed itself, and therefore no pregnancy ensues. This condition is sometimes called "luteal phase deficiency."

If the state of your fertility is important for you to know, the use of follicle stimulating hormone measurements on day three of your cycle is the trick of the reproductive endocrinologist. It has been noted that if FSH on day three of the cycle is already climbing (20 or greater) then the patient's chances of conceiving naturally are not very good.

If you are thirty-five plus, have decided you want to pursue pregnancy, and you know that you are not ovulating regularly, see a specialist as soon as you can if you fail to get pregnant after six months of having intercourse at the time of ovulation. You will need to pursue a structured plan to overcome fertility problems. Should you decide to use assisted reproductive technologies (ART), here are some of the options you will come across.

1) Fertility drugs. Clomid and Serophene are probably the most frequently prescribed. They are taken orally from the fifth to the ninth day of the menstrual cycle. They work by regulating ovulation. Pergonal and Metrodin are taken by injection daily until the middle of your cycle. Pergonal is LH (luteinizing hormone) and FSH, and Metrodin is FSH. They work by promoting the growth of the follicle in the ovary.

2) IUI (intrauterine insemination). Sperm are placed via a catheter directly into the uterus, where they have a better chance of reaching an egg.

3) GIFT (gamete intrafallopian transfer). Eggs and sperm are mixed outside the body, and the mixture is placed in the fallopian tubes.

4) ZIFT (zygote intrafallopian transfer). Harvested eggs and sperm are mixed in a petri dish, then fertilized eggs (zygotes) are placed in a fallopian tube.

5) IVF (in vitro fertilization). Sperm meet eggs in a petri dish, and when embryos form, they are inserted into the endometrium.

When nothing happens right away, it can be hard to sustain enthusiasm. "It stops being romantic after the first few times," one woman told me. "We were doing it twice a day for four days, and by the end I felt like, 'Okay, make your deposit already so I can go to sleep.' " The fertility treatments medical science can offer you are good, but they take time and energy.

It is not at all uncommon for a forty-plus woman to have many fertility procedures before she conceives. A patient of mine had three GIFT procedures and a ZIFT over a three-year period before she became pregnant. "By that time we had taken the pictures we'd cut out from magazines of babies off the refrigerator, where they'd hung for years to motivate us. It's funny, but when you hear that a procedure is one in three, well, you really believe you're going to be that one. I had a better grasp of reality when I decided to give it one more shot. We were giving serious consideration to donor eggs when I finally conceived." The rest of her pregnancy was uneventful and resulted in a healthy baby girl.

The pregnant woman over forty learns that her biggest task is staying pregnant. The risk of miscarriage is greater over forty, although we are not sure why this is so. But if you have early screening tests, and you don't have preexisting conditions like diabetes, hypertension, or obesity, you have an excellent chance of delivering a healthy baby. The best prenatal care you can get is key here, as well as eating right and taking good care of yourself.

## Questions Women Ask

*I was involved with a man for six years, and we never married. Now I find myself at forty-three wanting very much to find someone. Recently I met a man who has children from a previous marriage. I told him that it would probably be difficult for me to have children because I don't ovulate regularly anymore. He started talking about how he's always wondered what it would be like to have another child. I ended up resenting the whole discussion. I'm wondering if I should admit that I'm in transition to men.*

It's true that men can feel ambivalent when they realize that they aren't going to be able to have children with a woman they are deeply involved with. People in general would like to believe that every option is always going to be open to them and fear knowing some options are closed. You're forcing him to encounter his own feelings. Both of you have to accept that none of us can hang on to any one phase in the life cycle.

When he tells you he's disappointed that you and he cannot have children, it's hard not to take it personally. Try to realize that if you could have children, chances are he'd be ambivalent about whether he wants them.

One of my patients told me this, and I think it's good advice for any woman at this stage of the game: "If you're pretty much okay with what's going on, other people are going to be okay with it. I had two children and I didn't want more children, but when I found out I couldn't have them, I still felt sad about it. It was the sadness of saying good-bye to one part of my life. Once I got over it — and it was sooner than I thought — I felt relief and a sense of 'Okay, what now, what next?' When a man I'm dating tells me he wants children, my first thought is 'I guess he's not for me,' since that's just not my goal."

You may want to consult a fertility specialist to see if those doors are really closed for you. If so, allow yourself to go through a mourning period. The more comfortable you are with where you're headed, the more likely you are to find someone you're compatible with to share your life.

*How much should a woman really tell her partner about what she's going through during perimenopause? Is it true that men see women as less sexual at that point?*

Communicate as directly as you can. I mean, how can you not? It's not that he doesn't see. If he's close to you, if the two of you are intimately connected, and your periods are no longer regular, he notices it. If you can't sleep, if you are irritable and forgetful or having other subtle symptoms, he may recognize them before you do. He sees the changes that are part of getting older — he's seeing them in himself as well. It's better to include him in the process. There's this notion that if you share all of this with him he's going to be turned off. That really robs your partner of his ability to go through it with you.

If you're okay with it, he's going to be okay with it. If your partner appears uncomfortable when you discuss it, you may be communicating your own discomfort with the process.

To think that he'll view you as younger just because you don't mention the term *perimenopause* to him isn't giving him any credit.

*Is it true that an active sex life can offset perimenopause?*

No. But it can offset some of the less subtle symptoms one endures reaching menopause. Without intercourse, the vaginal tissues have more of a tendency to shrink and narrow, and they won't go back to normal if you resume sex years later. Keep in mind that sex doesn't necessarily mean something you have with a partner. Everyone can stimulate herself and simulate intercourse. And why not?

# 10

# MENOPAUSE
## How Will You Know It When You Get There?

Menopause is defined as the end of menstruation. It is confirmed medically after twelve consecutive months without a period due to a depletion of ovarian follicles (eggs). There are, of course, other medical conditions that can cause a woman to stop menstruating for twelve months. These include thyroid disease, abnormalities of the pituitary, eating disorders, too little body fat or weight (as is sometimes the case with athletes training for events), or serious systemic illnesses. But without the depletion of ovarian follicles, the loss of your period is not considered menopause. In the western hemisphere, the average age of menopause is 51.4 years.

Women in their forties who reach menopause often ask me if there is something they "did" to cause it to come earlier. With the exception of having a complete hysterectomy in which your ovaries are removed, which causes a surgically induced menopause, there is little a woman can do to herself that brings on menopause. Studies have shown that women who are smokers and even previous smokers can reach menopause several years earlier than nonsmokers. However, genetics is the key factor in determining when you will reach menopause.

Unfortunately, the genes for age of menopause are not as easily tracked as, for instance, those for blue eyes. Your family history can provide some clues, but the dates of a mother's or aunt's or grandmother's actual menopause may be difficult to ascertain with accuracy. As one patient told me, "I always figured my mother went through it when I was a teenager, about the time I got my driver's license. My sister howled when I told her that. 'Do the math,' she said.

'That would make Mom about thirty-four — and having symptoms for about twenty-five years.' My mother's period and her age were two subjects never discussed in our house."

There are other factors that may influence the age a woman reaches menopause. These include racial background, height, the number of children she has had, and especially if she has had any pelvic surgery that might have compromised the blood supply to one or both ovaries. Some patients feel that by suppressing ovulation through the Pill they can "delay" running out of eggs. This is, unfortunately, not true.

So how do you know when you're there? Let's suppose that you're in your late forties and you haven't had your period for five months. Don't automatically assume that this is it. In order to confirm that this lack of menstruation is the result of an ovarian receptivity (response to a stimulating hormone signal from the pituitary), doctors recommend a test to measure FSH (follicle stimulating hormone). It's a simple blood test. Here's how it works: In an average premenopausal woman, the production of estrogen from developing follicles in the ovary produces a feedback mechanism in the pituitary gland that diminishes FSH production until later in the cycle, when menstruation takes place and estrogen levels fall, thus initiating new production of FSH from the pituitary and starting the cycle all over again. In menopause, the ovary does not respond to the FSH. There is no feedback to the pituitary gland to turn off production of FSH. The pituitary continues to make more and more FSH to no avail, since the ovary is not responding. A high level of FSH is therefore what your doctor is testing your blood for.

As I mentioned earlier, FSH levels can begin to rise in the transition period into menopause despite a continuation of some irregular bleeding. Therefore, it may also be helpful to measure serum estrogen levels, usually in the form of the dominant estrogen known as estradiol. In true menopause, this will be low.

Paradoxically, in the transition there can be instances where the estradiol level comes back into a nonmenopausal range while the FSH has begun to rise and is reported in a range compatible with menopause. This normally happens within one to two years before the final menstrual period.

With paradoxical test results and irregular cycles, it's little wonder women aren't always exactly sure they've reached menopause. There are, however, two symptoms associated with menopause that most of my patients are familiar with: hot flashes and dryness in the vagina. Combine these with an absent period and a fifty-something age range, and you can be pretty sure you're there.

## Hot Flashes

Hot flashes are the most common and best-known symptom among menopausal women. What do they feel like?

*I start feeling warm. My pulse goes up. It's like when you've raced to flag down a cab and you get in, and five minutes later you start to sweat. Tropical is the word that comes to mind.*

*It feels like a blowtorch held up to my face. I seriously want to rip my clothes off.*

*Uncomfortable. A spreading feeling of warmth, mostly in my face and chest. Not awful, although my makeup runs, and sometimes my face turns so red people ask what's going on.*

*I was on a bus in the middle of winter when my first one hit. I had on a fur coat and hat. Well, off came the coat, off came the hat, off came the sweater. I even had my shoes off when I stepped off that bus.*

*Like you're running a fever. I was in the office, and I said, "What in the world is this?" It was like a wave of heat. I thought, "I've got the flu, and I've got it bad." But the women I work with who had been there before knew exactly what it was.*

Hot flashes can range from nothing more than occasional feelings of warmth accompanied by an increased pulse to nearly hourly waves of heat, drenching sweat, and racing heart.

They are often triggered by a hot environment, eating hot or spicy foods or beverages, alcohol, caffeine, or even stress. Sometimes there are no discernible triggers.

The hot flash (sometimes called a "hot flush") is actually a "vasomotor instability." When your supply of estrogen dwindles, the hypothalamus, the heat-regulating center in the brain, goes awry. It's theorized that when a woman's estrogen level drops suddenly, the hypothalamus interprets this as a drop in body temperature. It responds by triggering mechanisms to warm you up. Blood rushes to the skin. You flush. The sensation can quickly travel through your whole body. While uncomfortable, hot flashes are not medically dangerous to you.

These sensations may last anywhere from thirty seconds to thirty minutes. They can range from a few episodes a year up to three or four an hour. Although hot flashes may occur in the stages just before actual menopause, they are most prevalent in the year or two following menopause. In about two-thirds of women, they can last from one to five years. About one-quarter of women will experience hot flashes for up to ten years. A very small minority, less than 10 percent, may experience them for more than ten years.

Hot flashes seem to be the most severe in women who have a surgical menopause (surgical removal of the ovaries). This is probably related to the fact that the drop in estrogen levels in these patients is so abrupt and so complete.

Women sometimes ask me if they have "risk factors" for hot flashes. It is true that women with more severe hot flashes tend to weigh less and have less body fat. But there really is no relationship between hot flashes and age, marital status, number of children, age of first menstrual period, age of menopause, height, medical problems, race, or social class.

## What You Can Do About Hot Flashes

Beyond hormone replacement therapy, which is discussed in the next chapter, here are some tips for handling and countering hot flashes.

- Dress in layers of light clothing. One hundred percent cotton, which absorbs moisture and allows heat to escape, is better than polyester, which traps heat. Choose pieces you can remove easily, such as jackets and button-down sweaters. Wear skirts instead of pants, and summer-weight nylons.

- Keep your work and home environments as cool as you can. Warm environments can trigger hot flashes and certainly make them feel worse. A portable, battery-operated desk fan, available for about ten dollars at drugstores, can help when you're having thermostat wars with your colleagues at work, or you can't control the heat or air-conditioning.

- Keep a spray bottle of water in your briefcase or in your desk. Douse your wrists or your face when you feel that sudden warmth. This works quite well if you can't jump into a cold shower. Moist towelettes you can buy at most drugstores and keep in your purse can also be refreshing.

- Limit caffeine and alcohol. Both can trigger hot flashes.

- Don't stop exercising. Regular exercise can actually help to counter hot flashes. One theory is that exercise raises the level of activity of endorphins in the body, which may alleviate hot flashes.

- Stressful situations act as hot flash triggers for some women, so avoid emotionally charged or stressful events when you can. Many women learn how to cope with hot flashes and even to joke about them after a time, but when they first happen they can be very unsettling. If you can delay that major speech, the family reunion, the dinner with an old ex from high school that's been making you nervous, then go ahead and be good to yourself. Hot flashes are time limited. They will pass.

- There hasn't been a study that confirms that vitamin E helps to relieve hot flashes, but many women swear by it. The recommended dose is 400 IU per day. Don't take more than 1,000 IU — at that level you'll be very likely to experience tiredness and feelings of muscle weakness.

- You may have heard clonidine mentioned for helping keep hot flashes at bay. Clonidine is a medication for high blood pressure, but research has shown that women using it find it reduces hot flashes. It is not clear how it works to relieve hot flashes, and it is not as effective as estrogen in blocking them. In high doses, clonidine can cause dry mouth and dizziness. However, for women who can't take estrogen, clonidine, delivered via a skin patch worn on the shoulder and replaced once a week, can be very helpful.

- Bellergal is another drug that doctors prescribe to help women who are enduring frequent hot flashes, especially those who have breast cancer and want to avoid taking estrogen supplements.

    Bellergal is a tranquilizer. While it doesn't eliminate hot flashes, it can cut the frequency in half. It is theorized that this is because it has its strongest effect on perspiration.

    You are taking phenobarbital when you take Bellergal, although the levels are not very high. Addiction to the drug has not been cited in the literature as a problem because of the low dose.

## Night Sweats

Night sweats are hot flashes that wake you in the middle of the night. Women complain about waking up drenched in sweat, sheets wet, nightclothes soaking. Night sweats only last a minute or two, but that doesn't count the time it takes to towel off, change clothes, or just plain fall back to sleep. If you feel anxious afterward it's because your heart rate goes up and your body temperature rises. This is normal.

If you have started taking your pulse, as many women do when they have these symptoms, realize that it isn't unusual for the pulse to go as high as 150 beats a minute during a hot flash. (A resting pulse should be between sixty and one hundred, depending on your level of physical fitness.) A high pulse rate feels uncomfortable, but it doesn't mean you are having a heart attack. It will usually go down if you distract yourself.

The following are some tips for alleviating the discomfort of night sweats.

- If you're sleeping with a partner, exchange that king-size top sheet or blanket for two single ones. Yes, it will be harder to make your bed, but if you need to kick off the covers to cool down at night when your partner maintains that the room is freezing, you can.
- Keep your bedroom cool. This might mean thermostat wars with your partner. You won't be the first woman to point out that while

he can always put on extra covers if he's cold, you have no alternative but cooler air and ventilation to help your symptoms.

- Use cotton bedclothes. Anything else may make you feel as if you are waking up sweating in a plastic bag.

## Urogenital Changes

Vaginal dryness and/or itching is typical during menopause. These are actually expected and normal reactions to the absence of the sex hormones from these tissues.

The vagina is an estrogen-sensitive organ. As estrogen levels fall during menopause, there is reduced blood flow and nutrients to those tissues. The outer folds of the vagina actually shrink, the skin sags and becomes dry. The inside lining of the vagina, the epithelium, becomes pale and thin. This makes the vagina susceptible to irritation, especially from the friction of intercourse. In addition, the acid-base balance, or pH, increases, and there is a change in the normal bacteria in the vagina. This may result in dryness or sometimes a discharge (which may be confused for an infection but is not caused by bacteria), as well as itching and burning.

### Dealing with Vaginal Dryness

You might not be able to do away with it, but you can lessen the impact of vaginal dryness, especially if it's interfering with your sexuality.

- Don't avoid sex and think you'll come back to it later. One way to keep vaginal walls healthy is to stay sexually active. Sexual arousal produces some natural lubrication, even in postmenopausal women. Sexual activity, including self-stimulation, helps improve blood flow, which will help keep vaginal tissues supple.
- Allow enough time in lovemaking. When you make love, do it in a relaxed, nonstressful atmosphere. It may take longer for the vagina to become lubricated, but this doesn't mean that you've lost interest. Your partner may need to hear this. Involve your mate. Your symptoms may make your partner worry about hurting you.
- Use a lubricant. Astroglide gets glowing reviews from many of my patients. K-Y jelly, which is water based, can help during inter-

course, although it will not provide long-lasting relief of vaginal dryness. Newer polycarbonphil lubricants like Replens and Astroglide may last as long as forty-eight to seventy-two hours.

- Make sure you're drinking enough water to keep your entire body hydrated.
- Consider the use of vaginal estrogen creams. The next chapter discusses estrogen at length, and if you are considering this method, remember that the estrogen will get into the rest of your body, absorbed in your blood. However, the amount of estrogen in these vaginal creams is very small compared to the amount you get from oral estrogen or skin patches. In other words, you'll get enough estrogen to deal with the dryness in your vagina, but probably not enough to stop a hot flash.

Estrogen creams are an effective way to relieve vaginal dryness. Two of the more popular ones are Premarin cream and Estrace. You apply a small amount daily for about three weeks and can usually continue it once or twice a week thereafter. It is important that you don't use it as a lubricant before sex, as it can also be absorbed into your mate's body.

Estrogen (particularly vaginal creams) can actually reverse some of the menopausal changes in the vaginal tissues. Estrogen increases blood flow to the vagina, thus it thickens the epithelium, improves the pH balance, and reduces overall dryness, irritation, and painful intercourse.

## Changes in the Bladder

Normal aging as well as declining estrogen levels may result in more frequent urination and even "urinary incontinence," which is the medical term for the involuntary loss of urine, particularly when sneezing or coughing. Incontinence, however, is a complex medical issue. If you suddenly experience involuntary loss of urine, you should certainly consult a doctor.

The bladder and urethra develop from the same tissues as the vagina in the growing embryo, so it is not surprising that the hormonal changes during menopause have an effect on them as well. The cells lining the urinary tract become thinner and more easily inflamed. This may result in an increase in the frequency and urgency of urination, often without any bacterial cause — although these changes in the urinary tract can increase the risk of actual bacterial urinary tract and bladder infections.

Cranberry juice and vitamin C, either in pill form or from natural sources such as orange juice, can prevent urinary tract infections by acidifying the urine. Bacteria do less well in a more acidic urinary environment.

Each woman's menopause experience is different, with the greatest differences being observed between women having a natural menopause and those whose menopause is surgically induced. When you reach menopause, relief of symptoms that result from diminished estrogen may be your primary concern. However, there are long-term health issues associated with decreased estrogen. These include increased risk of heart disease and osteoporosis, and unfavorable changes in cholesterol. Let's look at each of these.

## Heart Disease

Heart disease is not a symptom of menopause or caused by it. However, it is a concern of women who reach menopause, because women are almost immune to heart disease before menopause unless they smoke or have diabetes, high blood pressure, or very abnormally high cholesterol levels. The estrogen that premenopausal women make protects against heart disease. Postmenopausal women, in fact, are more than twice as likely to develop heart disease as premenopausal women. Women who are premenopausal have a fraction of the heart disease of men. After menopause, without any hormone replacement therapy, women start to catch up quite quickly.

With midlife women as well as men, heart disease is the major cause of death. It is also a major cause of disability in older women. Unfortunately, many women are not aware of their level of risk. Each year in the United States, many more women die from heart disease than from breast cancer.

The fact that postmenopausal women are more vulnerable to heart disease undoubtedly has to do with how estrogen affects blood cholesterol levels, a major risk factor for cardiovascular disease. Total cholesterol levels of postmenopausal women are about 25 mg/dl higher than those of premenopausal women. Total cholesterol levels fall between 10 percent and 18 percent in postmenopausal women who take estrogen.

There are different types of cholesterol. The so-called good cholesterol, HDL (high-density lipoproteins), are believed to protect against heart disease. The LDL (low-density lipoproteins) raise one's risk of heart disease. In menopause, the drop in estrogen causes an increase in LDL and a decrease in HDL levels. This is thought to make postmenopausal women more prone to develop atherosclerosis, or "narrowing of the arteries."

In addition, it is believed that estrogen has a direct effect on the heart, acting as a vasodilating agent and helping to keep coronary arteries open, thus preventing heart attack.

Although all human beings past the age of fifty are at some risk for heart disease, there are factors that increase that risk. They include the following:

- Advancing age
- African American race
- A close relative who has had a heart attack or stroke prior to age sixty
- Physical inactivity
- High blood pressure
- Abnormal cholesterol levels
- Diabetes
- Cigarette smoking
- Being 20 percent or more over ideal weight
- Stress
- Drinking more than three alcoholic beverages daily
- Being postmenopausal, especially if experienced early (before age forty) or induced by surgery or other medical means

What can you do to reduce your risk? First, look at the list of risk factors and make a commitment to eliminating anything on that list that you can do something about. Next, have your cholesterol levels taken. After menopause it's essential that you get a complete lipid profile, which will give you not just your total cholesterol levels but your levels of triglycerides, HDL, LDL, and the ratio of HDL to total cholesterol. If you haven't reached menopause yet, have this profile done now, so that you have a baseline for comparison after menopause to see what, if anything, the lack of estrogen is doing to your cholesterol.

If you find you have an elevated cholesterol level, reduce the amount of fat and cholesterol in your diet and increase fiber. Exercise aerobically at least three times a week for a minimum of twenty minutes — preferably fifty.

What about taking hormones to decrease your risk of heart disease? In the next chapter I discuss that at length.

## Osteoporosis

According to the National Osteoporosis Foundation, one-third of all women over sixty-five will suffer one or more vertebral fractures as a result of osteoporosis (porous bones). Each year 300,000 women suffer hip fractures. The rate of hip fracture for women is two to three times higher than for men. Indeed, one out of every six women will suffer hip fractures in their lifetimes, a risk equal to the combined risks of developing breast, uterine, and ovarian cancer. Scientists estimate that the prevalence of osteoporosis will double by the year 2020 as the population ages. The cost to individuals as well as society is huge. More than $10 billion is spent annually on acute care associated with hip fractures alone. This doesn't include the long-term convalescent costs of nursing care, nursing home stays, or costs attributable to changes in lifestyle as a result of disability from a fracture.

### Understanding Bone Metabolism

There are 206 bones in your body. They give you support, they allow you to go about your daily activities, and they protect your vital organs. Bone marrow even manufactures new blood cells. Ninety-nine percent of the calcium in your body is stored in your bones.

There are two types of bone tissue. Trabecular bone consists of a network of bony plates resembling latticework or scaffolding that is lightweight yet extremely strong. This is found mostly in the vertebrae, the breastbone, the top of the pelvis, and the ends of the long bones (arms and legs). Surrounding the trabecular bone is a thin sheet of denser cortical bone. Cortical bone is also the major type of bone tissue in the arms and legs.

Although you may think of bone as inert and unchanging, it is living tissue and like all living tissue is constantly changing, breaking down old cells and replacing them with new cells (the process physicians refer to as "bone remodeling"). Your bone mass — that is, the total amount of bone in your skeleton — is maintained in a delicate balance between the breakdown of old bone and the formation of new bone.

Calcium is so vital to the human body that there is an elaborate system of hormones to ensure that there is always enough of it in your blood. The three hormones that mainly regulate calcium, the main building block of bone, are parathyroid hormone, vitamin D, and calcitonin. Calcium metabolism is also influenced by several other hormones, most significantly estrogen and thyroid hormone.

From the time you are born until you reach early adulthood you produce much more new bone tissue than you lose through bone breakdown. Around age thirty-five, however, one reaches skeletal maturity. Medically this is known as "peak bone mass." After this point an imbalance in the bone remodeling system begins, so that old bone removal outpaces the formation of new bone. Calcium absorption also declines with age. This becomes much more marked after menopause, because estrogen enhances the body's ability to absorb calcium. Estrogen also helps block the bone-dissolving actions of other hormones. Progesterone, a hormone that is markedly diminished in the decade prior to menopause, appears to help protect bone mass as well.

From age thirty-five until menopause, cortical bone is lost at a rate of .3 percent to .5 percent per year. After menopause and until about age sixty-five, the rate of loss increases to about 1 percent per year. This actually slows down after age sixty-five. Women can expect to lose about 35 percent of cortical bone and 50 percent of trabecular bone over a lifetime. Men will only lose up to two thirds as much of their bone mass.

Osteoporosis and its precursor, osteopenia (low bone mass), can lead to spine, wrist, and hip fractures in later years resulting from bones continually losing density and strength. Women lose bone most rapidly during the first five to ten years following menopause. Twenty-five million Americans suffer from osteoporosis, which makes them more susceptible to fractures.

## The DEXA Test

The DEXA test is used to diagnose osteoporosis and its precursor, osteopenia (low bone mass). DEXA stands for dual-energy X-ray absorbitometry. It is the state-of-the-art test measuring bone mineral density. Standard X rays are not much help, because you'd have to have lost at least 25 percent of bone-mineral density before an X ray would detect it.

The DEXA test measures bone at the hip, spine, and wrists, where most osteoporosis-related fractures happen. Often women who have reached menopause and are considering hormone replacement therapy are tested at that time. If you haven't reached menopause, most doctors agree that you should probably only consider this test if you have significant risk factors for osteoporosis. The following questions can help you determine if you are at risk:

- Have you had a complete hysterectomy without taking estrogen?
- Has your mother, grandmother, or sister been diagnosed with osteoporosis?
- Have you ever broken a bone from a mild accident, such as falling from a standing position, as opposed to something like skiing?
- Do you have a history of thyroid disease or have you been diagnosed with hyperthyroidism (an overactive thyroid)?
- Did you ever stop having your period for six months or more when you weren't pregnant — from being underweight, for example, or under stress?
- Do you smoke cigarettes or drink alcohol heavily?

- Do you have fair skin?
- Are you small boned and/or thin?
- Do you use certain bone-robbing prescription medicines such as cortisone or antiseizure drugs?

Any yes answer puts you at increased risk for osteoporosis; multiple yes answers cause the risk to rise geometrically.

A DEXA test costs about $200, depending on where you live. It is painless and quick. You lie fully clothed on an examining table for about twenty minutes while a scanner that emits low levels of X-ray radiation passes over you. It gives no more X-ray exposure than dental X rays. The test measures the amount of radiation absorbed by bone. The greater the absorption, the greater the bone density.

Your results are compared to peak bone density for young adults (to show how much bone density you might have lost) as well as to that of your own age group (to compare where you stand with others your age, sex, and size). The results are called a T score. Your T score is the amount of bone you have relative to a reference population of young, healthy, normal patients. Thus, almost by definition your T score as you age will be a negative number. It is measured in standard deviations (a statistical term) away from the mean. Up to -1.0 is considered normal. A T score between -1.0 and -2.5 is considered osteopenia, which means low bone mass, but not yet osteoporosis. T scores less than -2.5 indicate a diagnosis of osteoporosis.

There are other forms of X-ray bone-density-measurement tests that are cheaper, use smaller equipment, and can be used to screen just the wrist, forearm, or heel. The bone surveillance unit that I codirect at New York University Medical Center is involved in an ongoing project to evaluate the speed of sound and attenuation of sound as ultrasound is passed through the heel as a potential source for monitoring bone health without any X-ray exposure (although, to reiterate, the current methodology uses minimal X-ray exposure).

## Treatment of Osteoporosis

The best treatment for this disease is prevention. Consume 1,000 mg of calcium per day. Postmenopausal women should take 1,500 mg per day. If not enough calcium can be obtained through your diet, take a calcium supplement. Getting adequate vitamin D, 400 IU daily, is also important. Exercise, like brisk walking, will strengthen bones and also help the heart, muscles, balance, and weight management. Weight training and resistance exercises have the greatest effect on bone. And, for women at risk for osteoporosis, preventing falls that cause fractures is particularly important.

Although calcium, exercise, and vitamin D are key steps in the right direction, they cannot prevent osteoporosis as well as estrogen or the selective estrogen receptor modulators that have recently been released and are discussed in the next chapter. Until now, the only treatment for osteoporosis was estrogen replacement therapy.

More recently, a new compound of pharmaceuticals known as bis-phosphonates have emerged. The newest is one called Fosamax, which slows the tearing down of bone. Unfortunately, it is not an easy drug to take. One must take it immediately upon rising in the morning, with a full glass of water. One must avoid having anything to eat or drink, including morning coffee, and avoid lying down for one-half to one hour after taking it. Its main side effect is reflux esophagitis, a fairly severe form of heartburn. It is a good idea to take 400 IU of vitamin D as well, as it diminishes the bone pain that some people on Fosamax get.

Perimenopause is a time of subtle symptoms. At menopause the symptoms are no longer so subtle, and the choices of how to handle these changes become more complex. The next chapter discusses the most complex decision women reaching menopause today need to make — whether or not to take hormone replacement therapy.

## Questions Women Ask

### What is "premature ovarian failure"?

Premature ovarian failure means early menopause. The average age for menopause is fifty-one. The earlier it occurs, the more likely your physician will be to label it "premature."

*I am fifty-five and I have still not reached menopause. Should I worry?*

There are many women who begin menopause after fifty-five. Just make sure you have regular Pap tests and pelvic exams and that you keep a good calendar of your bleeding.

*How long can I expect to be in menopause?*

Generally what women mean by "in menopause" is having uncomfortable symptoms that occur slightly before and after they stop producing estrogen. Most of these symptoms stop naturally after twelve to fifteen months, on average, although there are women who report that they have symptoms for more than a decade.

# 11

# PLAIN TALK ABOUT ESTROGEN

Estrogen is the number one prescription drug in America. Is it the fountain of youth? The only real prevention against osteoporosis, wrinkling, hair loss? The bearer of breast cancer? The cash cow of drug companies trying to make money off of midlife women? What's the truth?

At some point in the next decade you will have to make the decision about whether or not to take estrogen. Although your decision may be years away, this chapter will provide information you need to make it wisely.

This chapter isn't the final word on estrogen. I leave the intricacies to those doctors who specialize in hormones. Think of it as a starting point. Chances are, if you are years away from menopause, what you really want to know is this:

- What is HRT (hormone replacement therapy)?
- What is the real essence of the debates for and against taking estrogen after menopause, and why is everyone talking about this?
- Will medical science be able to offer anything different or better by the time you become deficient in estrogen?
- What developments should you be watching? What's on the cutting edge?

## What Is HRT?

Technically, there is ERT and HRT. ERT stands for estrogen replacement therapy. HRT stands for hormone replacement therapy, which generally means replacing both estrogen and progesterone the body is no longer producing through prescription drugs.

When your body stops making estrogen, your doctor can prescribe pills, patches, or creams that will give you estrogen synthetically. The amount of estrogen prescribed is not really full replacement; it is actually only a fraction of the amount of estrogen that the ovaries usually produce. But it is enough to relieve you of the two major symptoms of lack of estrogen women come to see their gynecologists about: vaginal dryness and hot flashes.

Don't let anyone tell you that the symptoms of estrogen depletion go unnoticed. Will you know when it happens to you? My patients will tell you in one word: "Yes." You will notice something. (Unless you're taking low-dose birth-control pills, in which case you bypass these symptoms completely.)

For 85 percent of women, the symptoms of no longer making estrogen will stop within one year of their final period regardless of what they do. The situation stabilizes. The mood, concentration, and sleep disturbances diminish because there are no longer any small fluctuations of estrogen. However, the symptoms of estrogen deprivation, such as breast sagging, vaginal dryness, etc., do not go away. You can grit your teeth and ride out the storm without HRT, and many women do. But, in making your decision about HRT, realize that there are roughly 300 different tissues from brain to skin to bone in your body that contain receptors for estrogen. All of your most important body tissues contain estrogen receptors. When the secretion of estrogen changes, your health and well-being reflect those changes. Your breasts, skin, and blood vessels depend on estrogen to stay flexible and toned. Estrogen keeps the uterus, vagina, and base of the bladder moist. There are also many sites in the brain where estrogen receptors are found. This may explain forgetfulness, memory loss, and other annoying symptoms prior to menopause.

## Do I Have to Take Estrogen Even if I Feel Fine?

Women come into my office who are clearly menopausal, clearly making no estrogen. They are exercising, eating well, and doing all of the right things to stay healthy, and they feel great. But I have to tell them that there's no question that however well they're doing, estrogen replacement will improve cholesterol and be good for their hearts and their bones.

Estrogen replacement can help prevent heart disease. After menopause the risk of heart disease for women increases dramatically. Women who are premenopausal have a much lower incidence of heart attacks than men. After menopause, if they don't go on hormone replacement, women begin to catch up pretty quickly. If they do go on hormone replacement, they retain that advantage. It's no small benefit. It is estimated that 500,000 women a year die from coronary artery disease.

In the recent Nurses Health Study of 120,000 women, which took place over a ten-year period, researchers found that women who took estrogen after menopause had about half the incidence of fatal heart attacks as the control group. The reason? Estrogen replacement seemed to improve a woman's ratio of "good" cholesterol (HDL) to "bad" cholesterol (LDL). Women who took combination therapy, which included progestin as well, reduced their risk by 61 percent.

Taking progestin with estrogen also seems to prevent endometrial cancer. And, of course, estrogen reduces bone loss, which helps to prevent osteoporosis. If you begin HRT at menopause, your risk of hip fractures will be reduced as much as 50 percent.

There is little question that estrogen has positive effects on skin. While it won't turn back the clock, it helps preserve collagen, which keeps skin moist. A loss of collagen causes wrinkling and thinning of the skin.

HRT has been linked with reducing mild symptoms of Alzheimer's disease. Recent studies have also found that women on hormone therapy for at least ten years have half the risk of getting Alzheimer's disease in the first place.

There have been studies linking HRT with lowering the risk of colon cancer. Even tooth decay rates appear to be lower in women who take estrogen than those who don't. Still, more clinical trials are needed before these claims become facts you can count on.

In order to get these positive benefits from HRT, however, you have to stay on it. One or two years isn't long enough. At least seven years appears to be necessary. Still, with all of the good news about estrogen replacement therapy, it remains a debated subject among women and in the media.

## What's the Debate over HRT All About?

In 1966 a book called *Feminine Forever*, authored by Robert A. Wilson, a New York City gynecologist, was published. He wrote about women in their fifties with smooth skin, youthful breasts, strong muscle tone — all because they were taking birth-control pills containing estrogen and progesterone. The book promised women one way to halt some of the more unpleasant aspects of aging. Sales of the drug Premarin — a form of estrogen still widely prescribed today — took off.

So began the debate over HRT. A truckload of research on the pros and cons of replacing the estrogen your body loses naturally followed. Female hormone replacement is a multibillion-dollar industry. Today the controversy centers around two issues:

1) Is there a higher risk of cancer, particularly breast cancer, among users of HRT?

2) If menopause is not a disease, should women be taking prescription drugs — often for decades — in order to ameliorate symptoms that might be dealt with naturally?

Let's look at these two issues more closely.

### What Is the Truth About Breast Cancer and HRT?

Nothing frightens my patients more than the risk of breast cancer. While taking progesterone along with estrogen appears to eliminate the risk of uterine cancer that was reported in the past among women taking only estrogen, breast cancer studies have been inconclusive. Studies, sometimes published months apart, have contradicted each other about whether there really is a risk and whether the benefits outweigh possible risks. The most frequent question I hear from patients when I suggest HRT remains "Will I get breast cancer?"

The latest study published in the journal *Contraception*, which I've mentioned previously, was the most reassuring. Two hundred researchers brought together virtually all the studies ever done on the subject of the Pill and breast cancer. Those studies included data from 153,536 women from twenty-five countries. They found that there was no increased chance of being diagnosed with breast cancer ten to twenty years after stopping the use of the Pill.

Granted, the Pill and HRT are not the same thing. But the study is reassuring, because these are long-term results from a significant population involving pills containing a higher dose of estrogen than those usually prescribed for HRT.

It's a beginning, and there is more research to come. My patients who are in their fifties have been frustrated making a choice this important with such contradictory opinions and studies in the medical field. But there is good news for you if you are just reaching perimenopause. In 1995 the National Institutes of Health launched a $628 million Women's Health Initiative. This is a long-term study involving 27,500 women. In the HRT portion, half of the women are receiving HRT, the other half a placebo. In fact, the group taking HRT is split into groups taking different *kinds* of HRT, so this study has the potential to generate a wealth of specific information. The researchers will compare these women's rates of heart disease, breast cancer, and osteoporosis. The researchers plan to publish their results in the year 2005.

This is a study to watch. In addition, there are millions of dollars being poured into other research and drug testing. One thing is certain: You will have options and information a decade from now that women today simply don't have.

### If Menopause Isn't a Disease, Why Is It Treated as Such?

Menopause is not a disease, and one can make an attempt to treat symptoms like hot flashes and dry vagina without medication. It's the protective benefits of estrogen that you give up when you decide against replacing what you lose at menopause.

Given the pros and cons, it's important for every woman to consider her options and make her own choices. You need to consider your family history and your overall health. Women with suspected cancer of the breast, or liver dysfunction or disease should not take HRT.

If your doctor says you are a candidate for HRT, you need to weigh the risks and benefits. As a woman, you are ten times more likely to die from heart disease than from breast cancer. Ask yourself, "Does the protection against a fatal heart attack outweigh a possibly greater risk of breast cancer?" Is it going to be better thirty years down the road to have bypassed HRT when you fracture your hip? Twenty percent of women who fracture their hips are dead within a year.

When I prescribe HRT, it's after a long discussion in which I explain everything and help the patient weigh her risks and benefits. HRT must be tailored to meet the needs and symptoms of each woman with her family history in mind as well. It's important that a woman leave her doctor's office not just with a prescription, but with the answers to her questions and a treatment designed specifically for her.

## What Are My HRT Options?

Women often have the misconception that HRT involves loading their bodies up with hormones. The best hormone therapy will give you the minimum amount of medication you need for maximum benefits.

Estrogen is prescribed in three ways:

1) Tablets. Premarin, made by Wyeth-Ayerst, is the most widely prescribed estrogen in pill form. It is made from the urine of pregnant horses and comes in a wide variety of doses. The usual dose is 0.625 mg, although 0.9 mg is commonly resorted to if the lesser dose does not hold off symptoms. Chances are when you hear of a study on women taking estrogen, it was Premarin that was being researched, since it has been on the market for more than forty years. Other estrogen tablets are Estrace and Ogen. The usual dose of Estrace is 0.5 mg or 1.0 mg. Estrace comes from a plant compound, and Ogen comes from modified plant estrogen.

2) Skin patches. Estraderm, Climara, and Vivelle are the most common skin patches prescribed. They come from plant compounds. Why would one want to try "the patch"? A patient I'll call Helena began taking the lowest dose of Premarin at age fifty-two. She still complained of crankiness and waking up sweating in the middle of

the night. The next higher dose made her breasts tender, and she complained of being bloated.

Some women like Helena have difficulty finding a dosage of estrogen that stops their symptoms without causing other symptoms. These women are good candidates for the patch. Small round, self-adhesive skin patches are now available that deliver estradiol through the skin directly into the bloodstream. This "transdermal" release of estrogen is continuous and gradual. Because the drug is not taken orally, it bypasses the liver. When the patch was first introduced, doctors thought this was a great benefit, because the estrogen is not metabolized in the liver. However, the effect on cholesterol, whereby HDL is raised and LDL is lowered, is exerted in the liver. Women on the patch do not derive this particular benefit.

These patches are worn on the buttocks or abdomen continuously, even while bathing or swimming. They need to be changed once or twice a week, depending on the brand.

3) Creams. Premarin, Ogen, and Estrace are available as vaginal creams, which can be inserted directly into the vagina. Creams do relieve vaginal dryness, but they have a relatively low absorption rate into the circulatory system. This means that they usually don't prevent bone loss or heart disease, or provide the other protections of estrogen.

When a woman takes estrogen alone (pills or patches — not creams), the endometrium (lining of the uterus) grows and thickens. This can create a higher risk for developing endometrial cancer. This is why doctors recommend that women taking estrogen also take progesterone, which causes the uterine wall to slough off, eliminating the risk. The most widely prescribed progesterone supplement is Provera. You can take one capsule that contains both estrogen and progesterone, or you can take progesterone as a separate pill. Other oral progesterones are Aygestin, Cycrin, and Prometrium.

## HRT Regimens

There are several ways HRT can be administered. The first is known as sequential HRT. A combination of estrogen and progesterone is prescribed unless the patient has had a hysterectomy, in which case the progesterone isn't needed. I tell patients that estrogen is the "good guy." You take that every day. The progesterone is taken for ten to fourteen days per month in a dose of 10 mg per day, although recently we have been reducing it to 5 mg a day. Most women will have a withdrawal bleed on this regimen after day nine, ten, eleven, or twelve relative to the ten days of progestin therapy.

Unfortunately, a lot of women can't tolerate that dose of progesterone for that period of time because it causes breast tenderness and mood swings. There is a newer regime that involves taking a smaller dose of progesterone all the time. Wyeth now markets a drug called Prempro, a combination of Premarin 0.625 mg and either 2.5 or 5 mg medroxy-progesterone acetate (the generic form of Provera). With Prempro there's no buildup of the endometrium and therefore no scheduled bleed.

This newer approach seems to work better in older women further from the transition who want to avoid periods. In the beginning (the first three months, usually) there may be breakthrough bleeding. After three months, 70 percent of users have no further bleeding. But if a woman on this regimen does bleed, since there is no predictable cycle, examination often becomes necessary to prove that the patient doesn't have an abnormality like hyperplasia (precancer) or a polyp. The preferred exam would include ultrasound and saline-infusion sonohysterography.

A third approach being tried is a type of cyclical HRT regimen in which women take estrogen continuously and progestogen once every three months. They go two months without a period, then bleed during the third month, which means only four periods a year. The bleeding is usually a couple of days longer and heavier than with other regimens. This method of HRT is being studied for long-term safety, so it's important to discuss it with your doctor.

## What Are the Possible Side Effects of HRT?

From the estrogen, women sometimes get breast tenderness from fluid retention. It can also cause fluid retention elsewhere in the body. Some women complain of dark spots on their chests and necks.

Progesterone, as I've mentioned before, can cause breast tenderness, mood swings, constipation, and weight gain. Many of these side effects can be controlled by changing the regimen or the type of HRT being used.

## A New Option: SERMs — Selective Estrogen Receptor Modulators

Consider a hypothetical fifty-year-old woman. Let's say her mother, her aunt, and her grandmother all had breast cancer. But her father and his sister died of heart attacks, and his other two sisters both suffered hip fractures and ended up in nursing homes. Such a woman would be absolutely petrified to take estrogen (for fear of breast cancer) and absolutely petrified not to take estrogen (for fear of heart disease and osteoporosis).

Imagine a drug that acts as an estrogen for heart, bone, and cholesterol while being a potent anti-estrogen in the breast. With such a drug, whatever one's genetic and/or environmental risk factors are, they are diminished. Furthermore, if it doesn't stimulate the lining of the uterus, there is no monthly bleeding and no need for progesterone to protect against endometrial hyperplasia and cancer.

This drug actually exists. It is called raloxifene and made by Eli Lilly. It is marketed as Evista.

About 12,000 women in twenty-five countries have participated in the phase-three trials of raloxifene. Results after two years showed that the women taking raloxifene increased bone density by 2 to 3 percent. The group of women receiving a placebo lost bone density. Raloxifene reduced the LDL ("bad" cholesterol) and total cholesterol between 10 and 12 percent.

Is it safe? I helped Eli Lilly design studies using ultrasound to prove raloxifene's uterine safety. The method of uterine surveillance I designed used transvaginal ultrasound and then saline-infusion sonohysterography, thus going beyond the requirement of the FDA. Interestingly, the FDA would have accepted periodic blind endometrial biopsy as indicative of what was going on in the uterus. The people at Eli Lilly understood that blind endometrial biopsy, although acceptable to the FDA, would be fraught with error, especially if the drug caused polyps. My conclusion is that raloxifene does not cause any precancerous changes in the endometrium.

There's even some evidence that raloxifene protects women against breast cancer. During the first year of the trial there was a 58 percent reduction in the number of cases of breast cancer among the women taking raloxifene. At two years, it had risen to a 72 percent reduction compared to taking a placebo.

This drug is currently available marketed as a prevention for osteoporosis. However, I believe that I and many other physicians will prescribe raloxifene instead of existing forms of estrogen for many aspects of postmenopausal women's health.

If raloxifene doesn't turn out to be the perfect answer, other SERMs currently being developed and tested will. There is no doubt in my mind that ultimately these selective estrogen receptor modulators will make many of our current approaches to HRT obsolete. Again, your youth is on your side, and you will have many options that women who are currently post menopause clearly don't have.

## Questions Women Ask

*I'm doing great on Loestrin, but I'm going to be fifty soon. Do I have to switch to something else?*
The effective estrogenic potency of Loestrin is about double that of the starting level of traditional HRT. HRT contains less estrogen than even the lowest-dose birth-control pills. In simple terms, it takes more medication to stop ovulation than it does to replace estrogen in a woman who is no longer making any. Again, the goal is always the least medication for the most benefit. This is where a sensitive doctor plays a key role.

When a patient reaches age fifty or thereabouts, I can ascertain by serum FSH (follicle stimulating hormone) level on day six of the week she is on the placebo pills (recall that on birth-control pills, one week of pills are placebos) whether FSH has risen, signifying menopause rather than transition. If it has, I will usually switch the patient to more traditional HRT. This will give her the same relief from menopausal symptons as well as effective protection in terms of heart, bone, and cholesterol while diminishing any risk to the breast (if one exists) and for deep vein thrombosis (DVT). DVTs are blood clots in the legs and pelvis that in the worst-case scenario can send little pieces, or emboli, to the lungs (known as pulmonary emboli). This can be very serious and occasionally even fatal. DVT is a very small (1 in 100,000) risk of birth-control pills and HRT.

When women are doing really well on low-dose birth-control pills, physicians may wait a year or two after menopause before "rocking the boat" by changing the medication. There is always a possibility that the change to a new medication will bring side effects, and there can be diminution of the patient's sense of how well she is doing if she was happy with the first medication.

### Which is better, the estrogen pill or the patch?

In terms of treating most menopausal symptoms, they are about equal. Pills, however, are slightly more effective than the patch at providing protection from osteoporosis, and the patch does not have the effect on cholesterol (HDL and LDL) that pills do. Some women who experience breast tenderness or nausea when taking tablets find that they do not have these symptoms with the patch. Some women are shy around new sexual partners when wearing the patch, but it's easier to remember than tablets.

### How soon can one expect to feel better after starting HRT?

Side effects such as vaginal dryness, hot flashes, and night sweats disappear almost immediately, definitely within weeks for 90 percent of women taking estrogen. Trouble concentrating, forgetfulness, and anxiety are usually relieved within a month. HRT sometimes helps a woman's sex drive because it makes her feel so much better overall. Sleep problems caused by waning estrogen levels will also clear up, usually within a month. In addition, after several months on HRT you should notice less dryness of your skin and hair.

### How long will I have to stay on HRT?

Basically, the concept is to stay on these drugs indefinitely. Why? When you come off of HRT you will effectively then go through menopause, and you will begin to lose the protection of estrogen to the heart, bones, and cholesterol levels. Researchers studying estrogen and heart disease see the greatest benefits in long-term use. And to prevent osteoporosis, a woman must use estrogen for at least seven years.

Many patients are concerned about the prospect of staying on these drugs for the rest of their lives. I recommend that they come in every six months, and we can reevaluate.

> *My sister had a terrible time on HRT, especially the progesterone, and she quit HRT altogether. Does this mean that I'll be a poor candidate?*

It's true that about 10 to 15 percent of women experience PMS-like symptoms from progesterone that are bad enough for them to want to stop the drug. Many of these symptoms clear up within five months, though. You don't say how long your sister waited before she stopped taking HRT.

Every woman is an individual when it comes to how she will respond to HRT. There is an ever-growing number of medications and potencies available for use in HRT, and a skillful doctor can help you adjust the treatment to find the one that works best for you.

> *Is there any danger to just stopping HRT cold turkey?*

No. The half-life of these medications is very short. But within days to weeks after coming off these medications, the effects of lack of estrogen will begin in terms of the heart, bone, cholesterol, and any estrogen deprivation symptoms (hot flashes, dry vagina, etc.).

> *I keep getting a rash from the patch. Does this mean I shouldn't use this form of estrogen?*

Are you changing the patch on a regular schedule? When you change it, do you make sure your skin is dry where you apply it? Sometimes women have to try different areas of the body to find one that is not as sensitive to the patch. While you experiment, you might find an antihistamine, such as those in over-the-counter cold remedies, helpful in reducing the itching.

> *They say that no more than one in four women currently opt for HRT. Why should I?*

Much of this reluctance is unfortunate and dates back to the days women as well as their doctors believed "Hormones cause cancer." In those days, women took estrogen without progesterone and increased their risk of urerine cancer. Breast cancer wasn't the issue being discussed, but the word *cancer* stuck. An entire generation of women my mother's age were afraid to take estrogen, and their physicians were afraid to prescribe it. As more information emerges, I believe the number of women willing to try HRT will go up. There is a difference between women who take HRT for relief of symptoms like hot flashes and dry vagina, which disappear for many women in twelve to eighteen months anyway, and those women who are taking it for health maintenance.

### Do I run a greater risk of stroke by taking HRT?

The concept of the risk of stroke related to hormone replacement therapy is quite old and no longer adhered to. It is not dissimilar to concerns about increased blood pressure in the past. In the early days of hormone replacement therapy it was felt that women with high blood pressure should not take estrogen because they were at risk for stroke. This has turned around 180 degrees. Now women with hypertension are among the first to be offered hormone replacement therapy because of the tremendous benefits that HRT can give the cardiovascular system in terms of reduction of heart disease and stroke. (There is less estrogen in HRT than in birth-control pills, which is why HRT is recommended for women with hypertension and birth-control pills are not.)

### Occasionally I forget to take a dose of estrogen. Should I take two the next day?

When you miss a low-dose birth-control pill, your doctor will tell you that the next day you should double up. This is done because missing more than one pill, especially with ultra-low-dose pills, can (although it is not likely to) result in ovulation. In patients on HRT who are menopausal, there is no need to double up if an estrogen tablet is forgotten; missing a day will not change its effectiveness.

# 12

# GETTING SUPPORT TWENTY-FOUR HOURS A DAY

It's two o'clock in the morning. You can't sleep. You toss and turn so much your partner says it's like sleeping with a wolverine. You'd love the comfort of listening to someone else's experiences, hearing how she handles the challenges you face every day. Or maybe something is troubling you and you'd like some information, fast, to set your mind at rest so you can sleep. With a computer, a modem, access to the Internet, and an open telephone line, you can do these things twenty-four hours a day.

If you are willing to brave the Internet — and the World Wide Web in particular — this chapter will give you a map for finding some solid information and support. A wealth of information about all aspects of the transitional years — the psychological, social, and physical — is out there.

What type of woman uses the Internet to find information about a subject as delicate as perimenopause? "An enlightened woman," says Alice Stamm, who runs Power Surge, the largest support network and online virtual community for women in or near "the pause." Stamm is one of the pioneers of bringing the discussion of menopause "out of the closet and onto the Internet" through America Online and the World Wide Web.

"Let's face it, baby boomers are talkers. We like to discuss everything," Alice says. "When we start experiencing perimenopause, many of us need to feel support and camaraderie to help us cope with physical, psychological, and spiritual changes. Yet we're busy. We don't always have an extra evening where we can attend a support group. Power Surge is open twenty-four hours a day — and you don't have to get dressed and put your makeup on."

What brings women to Power Surge is a desire for timely information. In these days of managed care, when time with the doctor is often scarce, Internet resources like Power Surge can give you the right questions, if not all the answers. "It's always been my philosophy that it's *your* body — own it. Women can access the numerous newsletters, transcripts of guest conferences, resources, FAQs, links to other Internet resources, and reading lists. At their next appointment with their doctor they can have a discussion that's at a whole higher level. They can say, I read this about Premarin, or I heard that about natural progesterone, and I have these questions. We don't substitute for the doctor. We empower women to get the most from their medical visits and to be able to have an intelligent dialogue on the things that really matter to them."

The enlightened women Alice speaks about who use the Internet to get information about perimenopause and menopause are many. Her multi-award-winning web site has had hundreds of thousands of "hits" (web sites often have monitors built into their programming that track the number of people who log on). She has devoted regulars and a world-wide audience. "A good portion of what I know about perimenopause and menopause I learned in my travels on the Internet," Stamm maintains. And she's learned it from the widely known experts who are guests during conferences on Power Surge. "Women need information. The most many of these women's mothers have ever told them about menopause is that it would take ten years and be a pain! And the misinformation is out there, even as we approach the millennium. It still bothers me when a woman, say forty-four or forty-five, comes to Power Surge for the first time and posts a note saying she's just come from her doctor, who's told her she's too young to be experiencing perimenopause symptoms, and it's all in her head. I was doing a radio interview, and the reporter, a man, asked me what the difference was between a hot flash and an orgasm. Do you believe it?"

Later in this chapter I will tell you how to log on to Power Surge as well as other sites where you can get information and exchange ideas and concerns with other women. First, some caveats about going on-line to seek support. The Internet shouldn't replace your doctor. There is no FDA, no safeguards against false advertising or false facts. There's no guarantee that the person named Gail2 who gets into an intense dialogue with you about your menstrual cycles in a chat room isn't Joe Smith from Idaho looking for cybersex.

But if you're game, here is the best of the best, in my opinion. If you're an experienced web surfer, you have probably discovered more sites than I can list for you here. What I include is what's easy, what's informative, what's popular, what isn't filled with misinformation.

From the hundreds of sites, chat rooms, and databases out there, I used the following criteria in drawing up the list that follows:

1) No matter how good the site was advertised to be or what information was promised, if I needed special software to get there, beyond what one gets by subscribing to basic on-line services like America Online (AOL), CompuServe, Prodigy, etc., I didn't list it. Like many doctors, in my office I have access to the Internet through a major university. But I included only what I can access in my home with a solid computer and average modem.

2) I nixed web pages that take more than two minutes to appear on the screen, freeze your Mac or PC, or bounce you from page to page when you try to access them. Who has the time?

3) If a twelve-year-old couldn't sift through the site or read the information without a magnifying glass or a dictionary, I didn't include it. If you want to read medical texts, the library, where you can flip pages slowly at no cost to you, might serve you better.

4) I was wary of anyone selling anything — including expensive newsletters — so I left them out.

Things on the Internet change constantly. The sites and addresses listed in this chapter were current when this book went to press.

## Power Surge

This is the premier site for women who are in the midst of transition and are willing to brave the Internet. It was created and is run by Alice Stamm, quoted above, a New York–based freelance writer, editor, web developer and online media consultant, and mother of two grown daughters, who is best known by her online persona of "Dearest." Here you can "meet" other women in chat rooms, at cyber "conferences," and through reading their messages posted on "bulletin boards." Power Surge has won many honors, including Harvard Women's Health Watch, USA Today, and The New York Times Syndicate awards.

Thousands of women have discovered this site. These women are savvy enough to know the difference between perimenopause and menopause, Premarin and low-dose birth-control bills, depression and the blues. One of my patients posted a question about Loestrin and received E-mail from all over the world.

Power Surge has been Dearest's labor of love for more than five years. The fact that Dearest thinks of a hot flash as a "power surge" is a tip-off to how positive this site is and the level of discussion you will find here.

There is a library stocked with information you can download and read at your leisure. There is a newsletter you can subscribe to at no cost. Dearest fields questions from her online members.

If there is a book published on menopause, perimenopause, or related topics, without a doubt Dearest has had the author on-line, no matter how famous. If you can't tune in, you can read transcripts later in the site library. A word of caution: If you want to tune in when Dearest has a major author or physician on, get online and in position early. The site gets so busy that you can be shut out, like finding you can't get a ticket to a popular lecture.

This site is always active. The chat room is always busy. An avid and accomplished web surfer herself, Dearest is always scanning the Internet for new information, and she can find it in the most unlikely places. She includes an amazing list of links to other sites of interest to women, some just for fun (*Reunion Hall,* where you can find your old grammar school classmates, and *Found Money,* where Power Surge devotees have often found bequests of money owed them, are examples).

Dearest isn't selling anything, except maybe hope. It would be hard to find a more knowledgeable source on the Internet. She definitely gets two thumbs up.

How to get there: To get to the Power Surge web site, type

http://www.dearest.com. If you subscribe to America Online, use keyword Power Surge @ Thrive. It is part of Time, Inc.'s Thrive forum.

## Hot Flash!

Sue Spataro, a registered nurse who has done everything from surgical intensive care nursing to office nursing, first went on-line about six years ago when her husband, Joe, whom she calls "a real techie," introduced her to his passion for computers and the Internet. At first her goal was to reach other women who were also homeschooling their children to share resources. She developed Homeschoolzone, a web site that still exists today. Next she developed the Mom-to-Mom web site, a potpourri of issues that were of interest to moms.

Not surprisingly, a big issue was health. "There was such an outpouring of people wanting more health information, and it coincided with a time in my life where I was beginning to feel the first pangs of perimenopause. I thought, If it took me, a nurse, six months to figure out what was happening, how can other women possibly know? Back then there were no books on perimenopause. There was nothing out there. I had so many women subscribing to the Mom-to-Mom newsletter and coming to the web site. I did more and more articles about perimenopause and the health challenges associated with it, until Joe finally said, "Listen, you have so much information, let's move some of that off Mom-to-Mom and give it its own web site."

Hot Flash! was born. Her goal was to provide as much information as possible about menopause and perimenopause, and she does this fabulously. "I want women to hear about everything — hormone, natural, alternative therapies — as long as it has some scientific basis. There's not one therapy that fits all for perimenopause. It's important to be open-minded, for Hot Flash! to be a place where women feel safe and comfortable asking questions about what they are doing and what they need, without fear of being criticized for their choices. When it started to happen to me, I was looking for clear and concise information — then *I'll* make the decision. I wanted to give other women the same options."

Sue is also a freelance writer who writes for the *Charlotte Observer* and a frequent guest on radio and television shows, as she continues to get the word out about perimenopause. However, thousands of women "meet" each other each day through her web site.

The site has the smooth look of a glossy magazine and high journalistic standards. "I try to bring the latest information to the web site," says Sue. "I spend a lot of time working with health care providers to find the latest and the newest. Because I'm well-rooted in science I can find and understand information easily."

What's the most frequent question Sue gets asked about perimenopause? "The number one question is, When will it end? The number one complaint is: 'I feel like I'm losing my edge. I'm yelling at my kids. I want to smack my husband in the face for no reason.'"

Sue provides an environment where women aren't afraid to mention any of that. What else can you find on Hot Flash!? A woman who has never heard of perimenopause can find out what it is, what the signs are, what she can do to change her lifestyle, and what she can do medically. Women who are in the thick of menopause or perimenopause will find all kinds of fascinating articles and information about issues that are important to them, such as avoiding osteoporosis and heart disease.

A special bonus on this site is the handy "tools" you can download. For example, right now you can download a chart to list all your symptoms and what day of the month or the menstrual cycle they occur on. For no cost, you have an organized calendar to share with your health care provider at your next appointment and to help you understand your own patterns.

Hot Flash! is only one part of an interlinked site that contains its own bookstore, a site about younger children called Pitter Patter, a listing of doctors who have been nominated by their patients as "the Best Doctors in America," and more. Definitely a four-star site — and growing!

How to get there: http://www.families-first.com/hotflash. Don't forget to type the dash between "families" and "first"!

## America Online's Baby Boomers

This is a fun forum where you can find loads of information on all aspects of being a baby boomer. Once you enter the site, you will have to do a little scrolling to find a category called Baby Boomer Issues. When this book went to press, a hundred such issues were listed, including such topics as cloning humans, 20 years then divorce, new mothers, things I hate about marriage, and snoring spouses. Keep scrolling and you'll get to menopause-perimenopause. You may have so much fun reading the other issues that you never get there!

The menopause-perimenopause section is one of the more active folders, categories, or sites — whatever people call them. Here, women speak out candidly about their personal experiences.

Post your questions or suggestions and you're bound to get a response. You'll get opinions, feedback, an occasional doctor or two answering questions. You'll "meet" a lot of women who have just discovered that perimenopause was the problem after trying a host of ineffective solutions. This is a good place to connect and to learn that you are definitely not alone in this.

How to get there: You need access to America Online. Keyword: Baby Boomers. Click on Baby Boomer Issues. Scroll down the list — and keep scrolling — until you get to menopause-perimenopause. Click your mouse and you're there.

## North American Menopause Society (NAMS)

The North American Menopause Society (NAMS) is headquartered in Cleveland. They can be reached at 216-844-8748, or at NAMS, P.O. Box 94527, Cleveland, OH 44101. They have an official web site, however, where they post breaking news related to menopause, as well as fact sheets and articles you can download. Pretty basic stuff here, based on the most solid of research, but if you're looking for information and advice, it's an excellent resource. If you're tired of looking into a computer screen, they also have a Menopause HelpLine at a rate of $1.95 per minute (the average call lasts five minutes). That number is 1-900-370-NAMS.

NAMS was organized by Dr. Wulf Utian, a true visionary in the field of menopause. The organization currently involves a talented group of officers and leaders both in traditional medicine and humanistic approaches. I have been on their program committee and participated in their workshops and lunch conferences. It's a terrific organization. They are embracing the perimenopausal transition as an area of interest. Look for upcoming symposia, organized by them, on perimenopause.

How to get there: With access to the World Wide Web, type http://www.menopause.org. Their E-mail address is nams@apk.net.

## CompuServe's Good Health Forum

This is a place to truly connect. CompuServe has its loyalists, people who check in every day and "know" all the other people who likewise tune in often. But newcomers are always welcome.

CompuServe is struggling for market share against other similar services. I hope they will continue to do what they do best. There is a different level of connection here than there is on AOL, in my opinion. You may get back twenty messages of welcome from posting the simple message "Hi — I'm new here." The forums on CompuServe have always had that community feeling.

And CompuServe still lets you know when people have responded to a message you've posted on a bulletin board. You don't have to scroll through to find your last message and see if anyone wrote back. You may get private E-mail from people who are drawn to your story, but it is more likely that CompuServe members will respond "on the board."

Very active online self-help group meetings began on CompuServe. This is the height of being anonymous, and many people make active use of these twelve-step meetings where you needn't show your face. You can attend AA, Overeaters Anonymous, and others right from your keyboard by going through the Good Health Forum. It's even easier to get to these meetings by using the pull-down menu, selecting Go, and typing in Recovery.

All aspects of health are organized into folders by the "sysop," or system operator, so what you're looking for is easy to find. The sysop will often welcome you and send you a list of meetings and library articles you can download. How to get there: You need access to CompuServe. Choose Go from the pull-down menu and then type in Good Health. Click your mouse and you're there.

## Women on America Online

There is a link to Power Surge on this site, but you will find much more. Here you can find information and discussion about every aspect of being a woman, including perimenopause discussed from every angle. Relationships, health, diet, kids — you name it, and it's there.

One warning: It's a site you can go to and explore for hours without ever getting through all of it. There are great articles in the library on antidepressants, exercise, and diet. You may get so engrossed you never even get to the information on perimenopause!

How to get there: You need access to AOL. Choose Keyword from your pull-down menu and type in Women. Hit return and you're there.

## Medline

This in an online database of references and abstracts for 8 million medical journal articles from 4,000 publications. This is the place to go for specific articles and to do research.

How to get there: AOL will get you there if you choose Keyword from the menu and type Better Health. Better Health will also offer you online self-help group meetings. The address to the web site for Medline specifically is http://igm.nlm.nih.gov.

## SixKeys.com

This is coauthor Laurie Ashner's web site, where you'll find information about menopause as well as perimenopause. Here's a place to go for help with the emotional side of the Change. There are articles you can download on subjects such as how to fall asleep, how to reduce stress, and how to cope with depression. There is a wealth of material about building personal power and developing healthy relationships. The articles change monthly. The site also has self-help questionnaires and a motivational question of the day. Six Keys provides links with other sites that contain information about menopause or emotional well-being.

How to get there: http://www.sixkeys.com.

## 13

## YOUR EMOTIONS
### Mind-sets That Matter

I was explaining to a patient why her regular menstrual cycle had changed from three days once a month to two weeks four times a year when she smiled, shrugged her shoulders, and said, "Forget peri-menopause — I'm just hormonally challenged!"

Welcome to the world of today's transitional woman. What's out: feeling victimized or used up. What's in: resilience and flexibility.

Every day I meet patients who challenge the stereotypes and refuse to be slowed down by annoying, subtle symptoms of the change before the change. They waste little time on depressing this-is-the-beginning-of-the-end thinking. They want to know What now? What next? What can I do to feel like myself again?

Chances are you feel the same. Women of the baby boom generation have always set their own pace. If you're part of this generation, you walked into careers where women never ventured before. You fought to change notions about what it means to be a woman that had been ingrained in societal stereotypes for hundreds of years.

You may have delayed childbearing to an age where your mother had long since raised her family. With no role model for being a forty-year-old mother of a preschooler, you do it successfully and often balance a challenging career at the same time. Or you may have bypassed childbearing altogether and think of yourself as "child free" rather than childless. There are now 4,000 woman a day reaching menopause. The ramifications of reaching this plateau in the year 2000 will be vastly different than they were even a decade ago. A loud, collective, positive voice can't help but be heard when so many women share an experience.

Doctors see daily how important a positive outlook is to both mental and physical health. A woman's attitude toward transition often means more for her overall health than her estrogen levels do.

I meet women every day who go through the challenges of peri-menopause refusing to be victimized or discounted. They do what they can so that this transition doesn't slow them down. How do they do it? What do they know that other women should know? From them I've learned that the key to getting through this phase with confidence lies not only in procuring the best medical treatment but in possessing a positive and proactive mind-set. There are ways of viewing this passage that any woman can master.

## Knowledge Is Power

"I was scared, confused, ashamed, and feeling out of control. I felt self-conscious about waking up in the middle of the night anxious and having my husband say, 'Honey, what's wrong?' and then having trouble falling back asleep himself. I often felt like I would break into tears at my desk. I was so tired. But then I realized I couldn't possibly be imagining this. It just wasn't *me*. I became determined to find out what it was and what I could do about it."

In the case of perimenopause, ignorance about your body is not bliss. Your awareness can have a profound impact on your experience. Women who clearly understand their bodies, what hormones they are making and when, fare best. They have options. Even patients who choose not to take medical measures such as low-dose birth-control pills still achieve a sense of ease and control just knowing that these options are there if needed.

It's understandable that women don't always take medication or other proactive steps when they begin feeling the subtle changes peri-menopause brings. After all, the key word is *subtle*. When we experience symptoms we don't understand, the natural first reaction is fear. How you manage this fear is important. If fear is managed through avoidance, one grows more fearful and possibly misses out on the benefits of early medical treatment. If one learns to manage fear through communication and information, knowledge becomes power. Count-less times patients have told me, "I'm so relieved to know there is a name for this. I haven't been imagining it. I'm normal!"

Kim, forty-seven, is an active mother of three who has been on Loestrin for six months. "Looking back, knowing what I do now, it was clear what was happening during those fifteen days I was so out of sorts. It made perfect sense that my body was making estrogen, the uterine lining was building up, I didn't ovulate, and my body went out of balance. The funny thing is, I knew I was feeling low, but I didn't realize how low I was until I started taking these pills. I feel so much better, so much more myself. I'm reading the research; I'm watching my body even more carefully."

How does one turn knowledge into real power?

- Monitor your body. Keep records of your menses and your symp-toms. Bring them to your medical appointments. Report side ef-fects from any drug you are taking. Don't assume it's all in your head.
- Keep your eye out for information about the latest studies being done in the areas of menopause, hormones, and breast cancer. In 2005 the Women's Health Initiative study will report its results. This study has been following 27,500 women, half taking various types of HRT and half a placebo. Researchers will compare rates of heart disease, osteoporosis, and breast cancer among these groups.
- Carefully interpret the statistics you read. For example, if your risk of something is one in a hundred, and a study says your risk will increase twofold if you do this or that, realize this now means your risk will become two in a hundred. Chances are still ninety-eight in a hundred that it won't happen.

    Statistics are notoriously poorly explained in the media. If a certain statistic is troubling you, seek more facts. Learn the lan-guage of statistics. Talk to your doctor about it.
- Find medical experts who are comfortable discussing your doubts and questions. Never leave a medical appointment with a pre-scription in hand and questions unanswered.
- Thousands of women are working to bring national attention to

the health-care issues women alone face. Now that you need in-formation, it may be the first time you realize how woefully un-derfunded research into women's health concerns have been in the United States. But you and others of your generation can be a large, strong voice. Insist through your vote and your voice that research dollars are spent on the issues that touch you personally.

## Devise and Conquer

You've trusted medical professionals to have a health plan for you in mind, store your past records, and be familiar with them. In the days when a woman had one doctor most of her life, this made sense. But with the way we move from city to city and state to state, and change jobs and insurance companies, some women find they've seen ten or more gynecologists by the time they reach their forties. The person who must ultimately devise a health plan for you, know where you've been and where you want to be healthwise, is *you.*

Dayna, forty-five, says, "The doctor who delivered my child five years ago was great then. Now there's something different about him and his office. I get very little time with him at all. I know he still cares, but he's so hurried. It's like I blink and miss the appointment."

Katherine, thirty-eight, is a Midwesterner who found that her in-surance coverage when her husband switched jobs included a very rigid program in which she couldn't choose her own doctor or even make appointments without clearing them. She's learned to get the best of every appointment. "I was the type of patient who was afraid to ask, 'Is this gown open-back or open-front? Can I wear my socks? And what am I supposed to do with this sheet, wrap it around me like a toga?'

"I've learned to ask, to make some notes, to get copies of my records. Make no mistake: It would be easier to stare at my ultra-sound picture and nod my head, *Sure, I see what's going on,* than to admit that it looks like a bunch of clouds to me. It took a while to understand that the endometrial lining and the uterus are the same place! But who teaches us these things? Now that I understand what I'm seeing, I feel much more in control of my body."

It helps the doctor too. An enlightened patient who communicates isn't a threat but a bonus in making the correct diagnosis. Be a partner with your doctor in managing your health. Don't be afraid to challenge and inquire. And speak up when you're unhappy with the results of any treatment. It takes some women a full year of working closely with their doctors through trial and error to find the regimen of diet, exercise, birth-control pills, hormones, or whatever it takes to feel their best again. But you'll never get there if you don't speak up.

## The Glass Is Half Full

As you read this, menopause is probably years off for you. But not every woman is complacent about having the end of her reproductive years around the corner.

Melissa, forty-one, was surprised to find that she was in perimenopause at the exact moment she was determined to have a baby. "We spent years and thousands of dollars trying to get pregnant, but I was one of those women who became perimenopausal early, and nothing we did worked. There were things we could have tried, but they seemed so expensive, painful, questionable. When we'd spent twenty thousand dollars in fertility treatments trying to have a baby, that was the end for me.

"It was depressing to realize we weren't going to be parents when I was so obsessed with it. But one day I woke up thinking, 'I'm not going to have my whole life defined as a woman who wanted to have children and couldn't.'"

That was two years ago. Since then, Melissa's life has changed dramatically. She's taking a course in screenwriting. Her husband has gotten back into playing guitar. Since they felt that adults were important in children's lives, they became involved in tutoring inner-city children twice a week and coaching softball. They have started to see the glass as half full.

"If only" is a phrase that can drive you crazy. This is a stage in your life when all-or-nothing thinking is a setup for misery. What can you do if you recognize yourself as a person who tends to see the glass as half empty?

- Recognize that you may have been conditioned to think negatively. You may have no desire for another child, feel overburdened with those you have, but still feel depressed knowing that having another child is becoming highly unlikely. This is natural. It's okay to go through a mourning period whenever your life moves from one stage to another. But when patients can't get past the mourning period and concentrate on what they can't have instead of what they can, it's often because they've learned to embrace negativity as a mind-set.

Some of us have been around negativity so long that we fail to recognize it for the downer it is. A patient of mine, Eve, forty-eight, is a case in point. She told me a story about going to her parents' home over the holidays. "From the moment we sat down to dinner, my father trashed every relative, every neighbor, every person we know, and the whole family chimed in. 'Your uncle Alan — now there's a loser. And remember the people who used to live next door? I hear their son is back in rehab. He's worse than your cousin April. Did you see how fat she's getting?' Next came morbid monologues about the many relatives who have passed on and are no longer sitting at the table. And I thought to myself, 'No wonder I'm so negative.'"

Eve's father defines others by what they couldn't accomplish rather than what they could. He isn't going to change. She no longer joins in during family "roasts." When she can't tune her family out, she simply gets up from the table.

"I realize I attract negative people, like girlfriends with serious problems, or men who are depressed or need me to fix their lives. I used to think that bad things just happened to me. But lately I realize I've been drawn to people who think as negatively as I do."

Awareness is the first step. Eve concentrates more on what lies ahead than on what she has lost. These days she seeks out mentors among women who remain active and creative in spite of their challenges. She wants relationships with people who bond over more than their mutual problems.

- Don't be afraid to think positively. Some people have the superstitious belief that if they're negative, they'll ward off evil: "I'll think the worst, and then it won't happen." But is it true?

The belief that if you suffer enough in life you'll be vindicated is an illusion. It's usually based on the idea that things always even out in the end. Sometimes they don't.

There are plenty of people who think positively. The world does not come crashing down around them. Negativity isn't protective. It just breeds more of the same.

• Understand that chances are you still have more than half your life to live. Transition can be an impetus to make long-term plans and set goals, much as New Year's Day encourages us to plan for the coming year.

"It's a wake-up call," Jennifer, forty-three, told me when we were discussing some of the changes before the change. "I think, 'All right, I've had my time of being lazy about my health, of taking vitamins when I remember them, exercising when I feel like it, stuffing myself with fast food. If I want to be energetic and independent when I'm older, the time to get busy is now.' "

## If You Could Just Do It, You Would Have Done It

A patient of mine said it best, "You can't *just do it*. You have to live it. Three months on a diet doesn't work if you're just going to go back to what you used to do. You can't ever go back. And there are times when I think, 'I hate this. Why can't I just eat and do whatever I want?' But I can't."

It's frustrating. But when you realize that it isn't always easy, that you aren't a failure if improvement doesn't come immediately, you begin on a path to real lifestyle change and success that will endure.

Take it one step at a time. There's no reason you can't do it, but realize that it takes self-discipline.

Priscilla, forty-six, is a woman who looks better now than she did in her thirties and knows it. "I'm a few pounds heavier, but I'm toned. I have more energy now than I did then. I can run a block for a bus without feeling ready to faint."

She has what most of us want more of — self-discipline. Women like Priscilla learn that discipline brings an enormous sense of self-satisfaction. They don't learn it the first day. They don't learn it after one week. They want to say, "Forget it, it's not worth it" as much as you or I do. So, how do they stick with it?

- Build a healthy lifestyle one step at a time. Self-discipline isn't something we have or don't have, like blue eyes. It comes from the simple accumulation of positive experiences, of doing what needs to be done, step by step, even though it may be frustrating, even though we may be afraid. We start working through the feelings (*I'm too tired to exercise. . . . Sure, I smoke, but if you had my life you'd need something to take the edge off too. . . . I'll worry about how much calcium I'm getting when I'm fifty*) instead of trying to get away from them. In the end, the process of succeeding a little bit at a time builds strength and hope. That is what gives us the motivation to get up the next day and do it again.

  If you make a list of health resolutions on New Year's Day and by the end of January they're nothing more than a memory, realize this: Behind your inactivity lies an excellent, if not immediately recognizable, reason. Are you ready to move forward? If not, why not?
- Be specific about what you want to accomplish. Change "I want to eat healthy" to "I want to limit red meat to once a week." Substitute "I need more calcium" with "I will drink calcium-enriched orange juice every day."

  Keep your goals simple and positive. Too many goals are overwhelming, a good excuse for doing nothing at all.
- Don't tell yourself you are a lazy, worthless creature when you fail. Why hold your goals over your head like a cognitive whip? It only makes you feel worse.

  Believe that you're setting goals because you're worth it, that you can do whatever it takes to improve your life, and that it doesn't matter how often you fail if you learn from your actions.

  Because you had one cigarette doesn't mean you are a smoker again. You're a new nonsmoker, prone to relapse and in need of a plan to handle the next one. Because you've been avoiding getting a mammogram for two years doesn't mean all's lost. You're a woman planning to get a mammogram to protect her health, and you can pick up the phone this minute and make your appointment.

Discipline grows out of pleasure, the thought of the best that is to come. Discipline does not grow out of self-criticism. That only sets up what psychotherapists call "demand resistance." The more you demand of yourself, the more you resist.

Value yourself and treat yourself with understanding and respect. When you resist what's best for you, ask yourself why in an understanding way. What do you need to get yourself through your resistance? More support? More facts? A better vision of how you will benefit? More time?

- Recognize your fear. Fear is a common response to responsibility. Changing lifestyle patterns that you may have had for years to provide better health in the years to come is not only a challenge but a responsibility. If you find you're sabotaging your goals repeatedly, recognize that a fear of success can often reflect a fear of rising expectations: "If I achieve this, people will want more and more from me, and I'll never be able to do it all or keep this up." Set small goals and keep your thinking in the present. For example, don't dwell on the thought that you'll have to exercise every day for the rest of your life. Just exercise today.

- Gather support. Let people know what you are trying to do. Don't minimize the importance of support and reassurance along the way to any health goal you set. It can make all the difference in the world.

- Celebrate. Small successes lend the strength for bigger ones. Women who make necessary lifestyle changes without a sense of deprivation tell me they often feel healthier than they have in years.

- Make a list for yourself. What exactly are the pros and cons of making a full commitment to your health? What's meaningful for you? Don't kid yourself. A full commitment to health means some of what you are used to doing has to go and be replaced by new behavior. Self-discipline grows from a full realization of why one wants to change in the first place. It isn't a master-slave relationship with one's inner self in which you force yourself every day to do what you don't want to do.

Women who succeed realize that committing to good health is much more rewarding than worry, guilt, and regret. It's much more interesting than obsessing about what you should do and what you haven't done.

## Decide for Yourself

Every woman is a unique individual. Your health choices are just as unique. What works for someone else may not work for you. You have to take each choice as an individual one.

Kara, forty-seven, told me, "I remember times when my mother used to suddenly grip the kitchen counter and seem like she was going to faint. Those spells were probably perimenopause, but she never spoke about it. I wonder if this will be the next thing that will happen to me, now that my periods have become so irregular. But I figure all I can do is wait and see. Everyone who has gone through it tells me that each woman is different, so I'm going to put some faith in that. I know women who didn't suffer at all."

Many patients are often alarmed by their memories of their mothers' experiences. "My mother went into what we used to call a decline at middle age," one patient told me. "But that's what she expected to happen. She blamed all of her problems on old age. I think back, and she was only fifty. I consider that the beginning of middle age — not the finish line."

When a patient tells me that her mother or sister had a terrible time during the transition, I don't think she's wrong to consider that this could happen to her too. Genes are powerful. But it's also true that you can have an experience quite different from those of anyone else in your family. You have the benefit of medical treatments and information your parents simply didn't have.

Decide for yourself. Kara, for example, admitted, "My two closest friends are strict vegetarians. They don't see medical doctors but go to an herbalist. They wouldn't take an aspirin, much less a hormone. They know I'm on Ortho-Cyclen, and they are constantly warning me. But I have to live in this body. If eating less meat or taking herbs had cured me, I wouldn't be taking medication."

Another patient told me, "I really wanted to have my child naturally. I even considered home birth for a time. But as my pregnancy went on, it wasn't in the cards. I ended up having a cesarean. There wasn't any other way. I think it's going to be the same for me with perimenopause or menopause, for that matter. I'd like to do it naturally. But if I find that the symptoms interfere with my family life, my personal life, or my work, and I can't endure them without sacrificing something more important, then I won't be doing it naturally. You can't always have what you want."

Birth-control pills and hormones are not for everyone. Every woman's priorities are different. The amount of discomfort each woman is willing to tolerate is different. What you do with your body is intensely personal. You are the only one who truly knows what you're going through.

## Tomorrow Is the First Day of the Rest of Your Life

If you don't believe in yourself and know that you have the power to become the best you can be, why should anyone else? In my experience, there is very little my patients can't do if they make up their minds. The power of positive thinking is awesome.

Allison, at forty-four, was at the young end of the spectrum to reach full-blown cessation of ovulation, but she was clearly estrogen deficient and had only menstruated three times in over a year. An educated, energetic woman, she was hopeful the first time I saw her. She wanted a diagnosis that fit the symptoms that had bothered her for two years. I told her that her exam revealed that she was in perimenopause.

The second time I saw her, she seemed anxious and depressed. She finally told me, "I keep wondering, if I had taken better care of myself, if I had exercised more or eaten a better diet, this wouldn't be happening to me so soon. Right?"

Wrong. Science has yet to discover a way for women to keep ovulating or making estrogen naturally beyond what's programmed into their bodies, probably at birth. You haven't done a better job if you start perimenopause at fifty than if you start it at forty. The mind cannot control the manufacture of hormones or the number of eggs your ovaries have left.

Were there steps you might have taken in the past? It doesn't matter. What matters is this moment.

My patients tell me that when they stop dwelling on options they don't have, mistakes they made, or opportunities that have drifted away, they begin to see new opportunities. You didn't cause perimenopause, and you can't cure it. But you can feel better. You can get through this.

This time of transition and hormonal imbalance is something you can ameliorate but not totally control. Make it a priority to learn to live to the fullest within your changing body. Savor the rich life that is still ahead. If you don't see yourself as a person of enormous value and potential no matter what your age, who will?

# EPILOGUE
## Medicine in the New Millennium

Often the most healing medicine a woman walks out of her doctor's office with isn't the prescription in her hand but the information in her head. She understands what's happening to her body. She knows she's normal. She comprehends the choices she can make to improve her health. She isn't in the dark wondering, "What's going wrong here?" When it comes to the transition of perimenopause, knowledge frequently spells relief.

> *I don't panic when I bleed heavily for three days. I don't think, "Oh, my God, this is cancer." But I know what to watch for. When I pick up the phone and call my doctor I can talk at an entirely different level than I used to. I really understand what's going on in my body and why this is happening.*

> *It's a relief to realize you don't have Alzheimer's disease when you forget your computer password or a brain tumor when you get a premenstrual migraine. I never worried about things like that until I was hit with one unpleasant symptom after another and thought I was really sick with something serious. I can handle all of this now that I know what it is.*

If you're in transition today, you will reach menopause in the new millennium. What will that mean for you?

When I lecture to third-year medical students at NYU School of

Medicine, I start by telling them that things in medicine are happening at practically the speed of light. I tell them we use techniques today that in ten, fifteen, or twenty years will seem hopelessly out of date. These techniques will seem as archaic as making a slit on the patient's chest and placing a leech there to "bleed the bad blood."

They laugh, but I warn them that students like them will look at today's doctors in the not-too-distant future with puzzled, incredulous looks and say, "Amniocentesis? You used to stick a needle in the mom's uterus to find out about the baby's chromosomes?!"

When the process of cell separation is perfected — and I believe it will be in the next decade — a single nucleated fetal red blood cell will be detectable in the mother's circulation. The entire genetic component of the unborn fetus will be available.

Soon the human genome project — in which scientists are mapping out each chromosome for its genes — will allow physicians to obtain the entire genetic picture of the unborn fetus and perhaps even intervene at an embryonic stage to avoid serious debilitating and life-threatening disease processes like hemophilia and muscular dystrophy.

This is good news for pregnant women, but what's in store for you if you are in transition right now? Plenty. Think about how much we have learned and how far we have come in our lifetimes, medically speaking. Most baby boomers remember the President's Council on Physical Fitness. The program began with President Kennedy in the early 1960s; prior to that the understanding of the importance of fitness was anything but widespread. When my father had a heart attack in 1959, he was placed on strict bed rest for six weeks. After he resumed activity he was not supposed to exert himself. He did no exercise for the twelve years he managed to live after that point. Look how far we have come in our understanding of the importance of exercise in preventing heart disease. Today my father would have been advised to begin working out on the treadmill.

Doctors are often leery of making predictions, but I feel comfortable enough looking at all that is happening in medical research today to make a few predictions about medicine and women's health in the new millennium.

- Medical science will know more about how estrogen affects the brain. While research has concentrated on the physical aspects of estrogen deprivation, more research is now turning to the psychosocial aspects and symptoms. Estrogen's effect on the mind, memory, mood, and cognitive abilities are being studied avidly. Chances are some solid answers are only a few years away. You'll have much more information about whether you should replace the estrogen your body makes and the ramifications if you choose not to.

- You'll have choices for hormone replacement therapy that go far beyond what women have today. You'll be the first generation to be offered selective estrogens — medications that act like anti-estrogens on your breasts and uterus but estrogen on your bones, heart, and cholesterol levels. Raloxifene, a SERM (selective estrogen receptor modulator), hit the market first, but others will follow.

  I believe the understanding of estrogen receptors will continue to grow. The field of SERMs will expand. There may be various SERMs developed depending on which tissues are most important to your medical history and genetic predispositions. For instance, if one of your parents had Alzheimer's, you may use one SERM, whereas if there is a genetic predisposition for breast cancer, you may use a different SERM.

- The challenge of the next decade will be to recreate indefinitely in postmenopausal women the exact hormonal milieu normal functioning ovaries produce in younger women. This will require an understanding of what other substances may be involved and in what levels. Taking it one step further, if some of the "natural" ovarian hormone production proves to be detrimental (like estrogen is said to be for your breasts or unopposed estrogen for your uterus), then the concept of SERMs may allow us to do better than nature itself.

- You will have a solid thumbs up or thumbs down on many of the herbal treatments recommended for medical ailments, including menstrual complaints. Research teams are not waiting for the FDA to run their own tests when so many women are taking these remedies. They are conducting their own double-blind tests. Major universities in the United States are in the midst of studies in which women with perimenopausal symptoms have been given an herb or a placebo without knowing which they are taking. These women are being monitored closely. We'll see how these remedies stand up to the scientific method. When and if they do, doctors will have more alternatives to offer patients.

- Centers in the brain that control compulsive behaviors, such as overeating or the tendency toward addiction, will be delineated. The neurotransmitters in the brain will be better understood and better controlled through medicine. Mood swings, depression, and insomnia, which occur at perimenopause, will also be much better understood.

- If you think looking old and dry is a natural part of aging, you have only to look at the research that brought us alpha-hydroxy acids and Retin-A. You may find that you look better at sixty than any generation before you if the hundreds of medical research teams focused on understanding the aging process succeed in learning how we can oppose its physical effects.

- Your basic gynecological exam will change. I believe that vaginal ultrasound imaging will be part of every pelvic examination. No longer will a doctor blindly feel internal organs in an attempt to determine whether everything is normal. Already practitioners like myself who use ultrasound on a regular basis get not only instantaneous pictures of anatomic structures but also information about their functioning.

I have seen prototypes of equipment that will be to the current ultrasound machines what the laptop is to the desktop computer. They will be small handheld devices. There will be one in each exam room, or the gynecologist may carry the probe from room to room, not unlike an internist does with his stethoscope. Think of fetal monitoring. Twenty-five years ago they listened with a stethoscope to the baby's heart every fifteen minutes during labor. Now virtually every delivery in every hospital throughout the country has continuous fetal monitoring.

I even predict that the day may come when each patient will

have at home a device not unlike a tampon in appearance that can be inserted in the vagina and plugged into a modem. The physician on the other end will be able to image the pelvis without the patient's having to travel to the doctor's office. It will be the "house call" of the new millennium.

When I think of the ramifications of this, I think of the patient who is one day shy of being seven weeks pregnant and who starts spotting that morning. She's scared to death that she's having a miscarriage. She calls me and I tell her to come in right away. It takes major juggling of her preschooler and her work schedule to get her to the office for a ten A.M. appointment. She has her answer in three seconds, the time it takes me to put an ultrasound probe in the vagina. Both of us can see a quarter-inch embryo with a beating heart, very normal in appearance. She's fine. The embryo's fine. We both think that it's too bad she had to come all the way to my office for this.

With the electronic house call, women may no longer have to wait through hours of worry until they can get an appointment to know what their gynecological symptoms mean. Given managed care, that's no small deal. Women will simply modem in their pictures and doctors will diagnose them. Sounds far-fetched? Consider that the pocket calculator, the PC, the hand-held hair dryer, didn't exist in our youth.

- You will live longer. Life expectancy has gone up dramatically in the last 150 years because of things that we take for granted, such as vaccines, antibiotics, and water purification systems. High-tech medical procedures such as coronary artery bypass and hip replacement have contributed somewhat, but to a lesser extent, to this increase in longevity.

As we whirl past the year 2000, life expectancy will continue to grow. But the emphasis will shift toward improving quality of life — not simply longevity but vitality. Concerns about humanistic and holistic approaches and the ability to marry these with modern medical science will increase. Modern medical science need not be at odds with a more humane, compassionate, spiritual approach to people, their lives, and their health. I predict that traditional medicine will merge with the best of natural remedies. Doctors will know when nature does it best, and when to leave it alone entirely. Naturalists will understand that there are times we must circumvent nature to do what's best for the patient.

- Menopause may not mean you can't give birth to a child. I predict that women over fifty will have more children through various forms of assisted reproductive technologies. The science is in place. Donor eggs from younger women can be inseminated by your partner and then reimplanted into your uterus, which has been made hormonally responsive to the fertilized egg. Thus you can bear a child naturally who has your husband's genetic makeup. The future may bring the ability to inject some form of your DNA into a donor egg so that women over fifty can have babies that are genetically theirs and their partners'. Just as baby-boom women were once at the center of the debate about whether they should prevent conception, they will be at the center of the debate about whether to continue it indefinitely.

- There will be less invasive surgery. Most gynecological procedures will be done endoscopically through the laparoscope and hystero-scope — surgical procedures that use a thin scope to view the internal organs.

- I predict that menopause as a psychological concept won't have nearly the negative connotation it's had in the past. It won't be seen as the end of anything but simply the beginning of a new phase. With women living thirty, forty, fifty years post menopause, "the change" may become a signal of freedom rather than depletion, a time for oneself rather than a time focused so fully on others. By the year 2025 there will be two sixty-five-year-old people for every teenager. The definition of *old* will continue to change.

Perimenopause can be a time of uncomfortable imbalance. But it's also a signal that you have the time to do things preventatively that you can't do later on. Your youth is on your side. You can take control of the effects of the change before the change so that it is a much smoother passage. If you focus your efforts on health planning and leading a healthy lifestyle, I believe that at eighty-five you will have every chance of being like the sixty-five-year-old women of today. The issue will not be longevity, but the quality of your later years. It will be possible to stay mentally and physically vibrant, flexible, and active through knowledge, understanding, healthy planning, and wise choices.

# APPENDIX

## Diagnostic Ultrasound Images from Patients with Abnormal Bleeding

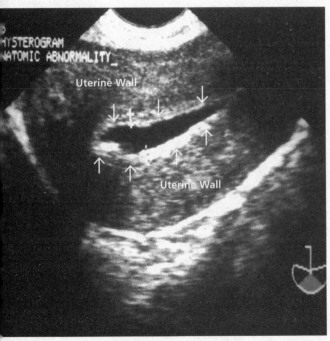

(FIGURE 1) This patient has a normal uterus with normal myometrial textures and thin, regular endometrial surface measuring 1.9 and 2.0 mm anterior and posterior wall respectively. The black area in the center is the fluid that has been instilled. This patient has no anatomic abnormality, and thus her bleeding is hormonally caused. This is medically known as "dysfunctional uterine bleeding" and by laypeople as "hormone imbalance." This woman does not need a biopsy, a D&C, or a hysteroscopy, and can be sucessfully diagnosed with ultrasound and saline-infusion sonohysterography. Small arrows depict thin, smooth, homogenous normal tissue lining the uterus. The uterine wall is labeled.

(FIGURE 2) This patient has a polyp. It measures 2.1 cm and is located at the top of the uterus. (You can see the outline of the Goldstein catheter halfway up the endometrial cavity.) The tissue surrounding the cavity is thin. This patient needs a D&C for *therapy*, not for diagnosis. Small arrows show the thin, normal lining of the uterus. The uterine wall (musculature) is labeled, as are the polyp and the catheter.

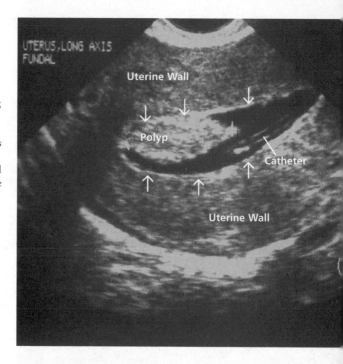

(FIGURE 3) This patient has a fibroid. This is a benign tumor of smooth muscle and connective tissue that arises in the wall of the uterus. Compare the black fluid outline shape in this patient with the previous two. This requires special instrumentation known as a resectoscope at the time of D&C hysteroscopy, whereby a wire loop attached to an electric current can be put into the endometrial cavity under direct vision and actually shave the fibroid away. This requires special expertise, but preoperative diagnosis means the patient can avoid an old-fashioned open-surgery myomectomy. Open arrows depict normal lining tissue. The fibroid tumor is marked.

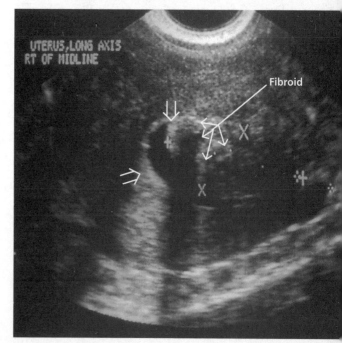

(FIGURE 4) This patient has fluffy white tissue (multiple small arrows) along the front wall of the uterus. This is advanced precancer. The tissue along the back wall of the uterus (open arrows) is normal. A biopsy done in the office would have a hit-or-miss chance of obtaining the right tissue to make this diagnosis.

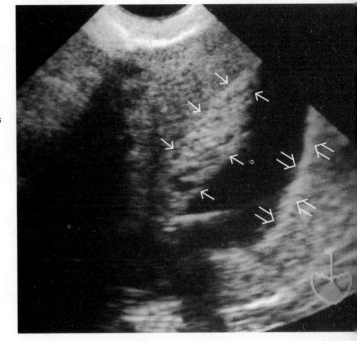

## Ultrasound Images from Premenopausal and Postmenopausal Patients

(FIGURE 5) A vaginal sonogram showing the lining of the uterus (indicated by arrows) in a premenopausal patient prior to ovulation. Notice the central thin white line surrounded on each side by two black stripes, followed by another thin white layer. This multilayered appearance is caused by estrogenic stimulation and is typical prior to ovulation.

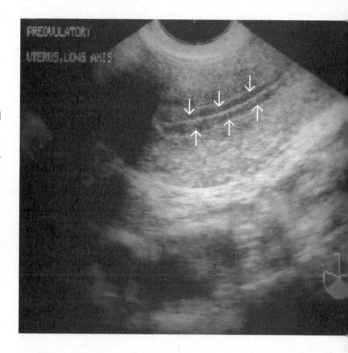

(FIGURE 6) The left ovary of the same patient. The prominent black circle in the center, which measures 20 mm, is known as a "dominant follicle" and is shown just prior to rupture (ovulation). The smaller black circles (indicated by arrows) are follicles that contain eggs but will not rupture.

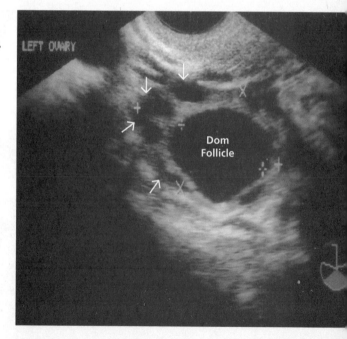

(FIGURE 7) This is a vaginal ultrasound showing the thin white "pencil line" lining (indicated by arrows) of the uterine cavity in a patient who is one year post menopause. There is no stimulation (buildup) of the lining because this patient no longer makes estrogen.

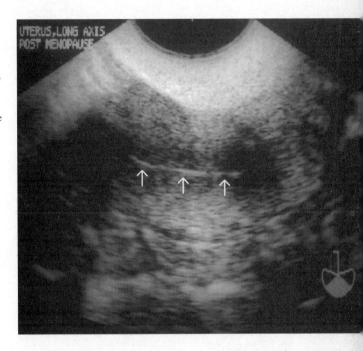

(FIGURE 8) The left ovary of the patient in the previous picture. It has no small black circles (follicles), as one would expect in a patient who is postmenopausal. The large arrow marks a large vein beneath the ovary. The ovary is outlined by small arrows.

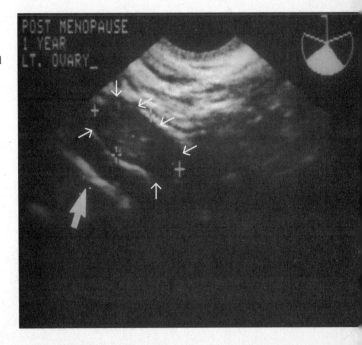

# INDEX

abnormal bleeding, 23, 29, 59, 120–122.
  *See also* dilation and curettage (D&C)
age, perimenopause and, 19–20, 21, 22,
  172–173
alcohol use
  breast cancer and, 130
  cholesterol levels and, 145
  cirrhosis and, 27
  hot flashes and, 175, 176
  libido and, 156–157
  migraines and, 40, 115
  osteoporosis and, 67
  side effects, 41
  sleep disturbances and, 41, 106
Alesse, 58
allergy pills, 37, 38
Alzheimer's disease, 36, 189, 190, 224
anemia, 55, 126
anovulation. *See* ovulation
antibiotics, 155
antidepressants, 32, 50–51, 113–114, 155
antihistamines, 37, 154–155
antihypertensives, 157
anxiety
  causes, 15, 41
  libido, loss of, 163
  mood swings and, 38
  symptoms, 35
  treatment, 109–111
appetite, increased, 117
aspirin, 31, 40, 115
assisted reproductive technology (ART),
  168, 227

Astroglide, 158, 178–179
Ativan, 109
Aygestin, 194

basal body temperature, 17
Bellergal, 114–115, 177
benzodiazepines, 109
bimanual examinations, 141–143
birth-control pills (BCPs). *See also* cycle
    regulators
  alternatives to, 59–60, 66–67
  benefits of, 54, 115
  breast cancer and, 57–58
  future developments, 60–61
  medical care while taking, 58–59
  menstrual changes and, 25, 32, 55
  myths about, 49, 173
  side effects, 55–57, 62, 156
  types, 53
bisphosphonates, 186
black cohosh (*Cimicifuga racemosa,*
    squawroot), 70, 73–74
black snakeroot, 73
bladder, urinary, 126, 179–180
bleeding, vaginal. *See* abnormal bleeding;
    menstrual cycle
bloating. *See* fluid retention
blood pressure, high, 56, 67, 80, 157, 200
blood-sugar levels, low, 14, 117
blood tests
  breast cancer, 133
  FSH, 18–19, 64, 147, 173, 197
blue cohosh (*Caulophyllum thalictroides*), 75

body fat level, menstruation and, 28, 45, 101

body weight
dieting, side effects of, 32, 38
hormone replacement therapy and, 196
perimenopause and, 10, 15, 21, 87–98, 172
questions about, 101–102

bone density, 28, 55. *See also* osteoporosis

botanical remedies. *See* natural remedies

BRCA 1 and BRCA 2, 133

breast cancer
blood tests for, 133
HRT and, 191–193, 197
incidence, 129
natural remedies and, 71
risk factors for, 57–58, 129–130, 133
symptoms, 34
treatment, 130–131

breast disease, benign, 54

breast self-examinations, 67, 130, 146

breast soreness, 34–35, 106, 195, 196

bromides, 106

caffeine
hot flashes and, 175, 176
migraine headaches and, 115
osteoporosis and, 66
side effects, 38, 41
sleep disturbances and, 106

calcium, 67, 97–98, 182, 186

cancer. *See also* breast cancer; endometrial (uterine) cancer
cervical, 135, 147–150
menopause, age of onset and, 21
prevention, BCPs and, 53, 54
symptoms, 30

cardiovascular disease. *See* heart disease

cervical cancer, 135, 147–150

cervical mucus, 17, 55

cervix, 168

chasteberry *(Vitex agnus-castus)*, 77–78

checkups. *See* medical care

Chinese angelica root, 72

chocolate, 40, 66–67, 115

cholesterol, 146–147, 159, 180–182, 190, 196

Climara, 193

Clomid, 168

clonidine, 176–177

clumsiness, 117

cluster headaches, 39–40

collagen, 190

colposcopy, 148, 149, 150

communication, importance of, 163–164, 171

Compazine, 115

concentrating, difficulty, 15, 21, 36–37

constipation, 105, 196

contraception. *See* birth-control pills (BCPs)

coronary artery disease. *See* heart disease

corpus luteum, 13–14

cramps, painful, 33–34, 115

creams, vaginal estrogen, 179, 194

Crinone, 60–61

cycle regulators, 21, 46–67, 83

Cycrin, 60, 194

cystic mastitis, 106

deep vein thrombosis (DVT), 198

depression
causes, 15, 42–43
incidence of, 22
mood swings and, 38
treatment, 111–114

DEXA. *See* dual-energy X-ray absorbitometry (DEXA)

diabetes, 29

diarrhea, 34, 105

dieting. *See* body weight

dilation and curettage (D&C), 118–120, 122–123, 131–132, 134

dizziness, 43–44, 117

doctor's visits. *See* medical care

dong quai *(Angelica sinesis)*, 72–73

dopamine, 38

dual-energy X-ray absorbitometry (DEXA), 184–185

dysfunctional uterine bleeding. *See* abnormal bleeding

dysmenorrhea, 33–34, 115

dysthymia, 112, 113

ectopic pregnancy, 54

endometrial ablation, 131

endometrial biopsy, 121

endometrial (uterine) cancer
causes, 28, 101
prevention, 54, 190
progesterone and, 60

symptoms, 29, 30, 120
treatment, 123–124
endometriosis, 30, 33
endorphins, 176
essential fatty acids, 79
Estrace, 179, 193, 194
Estraderm, 193
estradiol, 18–19, 173
Estratest, 158, 159
estriol, 18
estrogen. *See also* birth-control pills (BCPs);
perimenopause
adipose tissue and, 28, 45, 101
blood tests for, 18–19
bone density and, 28, 97, 183, 190
brain receptors for, 36, 115
breast soreness and, 34
cholesterol levels and, 146
depletion, symptoms of, 26, 189
menstrual cycle and, 13–14
unopposed, symptoms of, 12, 14–17, 36,
157
vaginal creams, 179, 194
estrogen replacement therapy (ERT)
benefits of, 186, 189–191, 197–198
defined, 188–189
regimens for, 193–194
side effects, 32, 195
estrone, 18, 101
evening primrose oil, 79–80
Evista, 196–197. *See also* raloxifene.
exercise
cholesterol levels and, 146
extreme, menstruation and, 27–28,
32
flexibility training, 95–97
importance of, 66, 90–94, 101, 106,
111, 176
strength training, 96, 98, 186

faintness, 26, 43–44
fallopian tubes, 13, 55, 168
fatigue, 10
fertility, 167–170
fibroids (myomas or leiomyomas)
BCPs and, 56
sizing of, 134
symptoms, 30, 33, 44, 120
treatment, 124–127
flaxseed oil, 76–77

fluid retention, 62, 105–106. *See also* salt
intake
follicles, ovarian, 13, 172
follicle stimulating hormone (FSH)
blood tests for, 18–19, 64, 147, 173, 197
fertility drugs and, 168
menstrual cycle and, 13–14
perimenopause and, 18
forgetfulness, 10, 35–36, 115–116
Fosamax, 98, 186
free-floating anxiety. *See* anxiety
FSH. *See* follicle stimulating hormone (FSH)

gamete intrafallopian transfer (GIFT), 169
gamma linolenic acid (GLA), 79
generalized anxiety disorder, 41–42
genetics, perimenopause and, 20–21,
172–173
GIFT. *See* gamete intrafallopian transfer
(GIFT)
ginseng *(Panax schinseng)*, 75–76

Halcion, 35
HDL. *See* high-density lipoprotein (HDL)
headaches, 38–40, 95, 114–115
health maintenance organizations (HMOs),
136
heart disease
causes, 180–181
prevention, 49, 190, 193
risk factors for, 181
symptoms of, 44
herbal medicine. *See* natural remedies
herpes, 32, 135
high blood pressure. *See* blood pressure, high
high-density lipoprotein (HDL), 146–147,
159, 181–182, 190
hippocampus, 36, 115
HMOs. *See* health maintenance
organizations (HMOs)
hormone replacement therapy (HRT). *See
also* estrogen replacement therapy
(ERT)
benefits of, 37
breast cancer and, 57
debate over, 191–193
defined, 188–189
questions about, 197–200
regimens for, 193–197
side effects, 195–196

hormones, 21, 88–89, 183. *See also*
    estrogen; progesterone
hot flashes
    causes, 18, 65, 174–175
    incidence of, 22
    insomnia and, 40–41
    treatment, 175–177
HRT. *See* hormone replacement therapy
    (HRT)
human papilloma virus (HPV), 150
hyperplasia (precancer)
    about, 128
    causes, 12, 101
    HRT and, 197
    symptoms, 29, 30, 120
hypothalamus, 30, 175
hysterectomy
    avoiding unnecessary, 123–124, 135
    risk factors for, 132
    types, 134–135
hysteroscopy, 121, 122–123, 131

incontinence, urinary, 179–180
infertility, 167–170
insomnia. *See* sleep disturbances
insulin, 28
Internet, as menopause information source,
    201–209
intrauterine insemination (IUI), 169
in vitro fertilization (IVF), 169
iron-deficiency anemia, 55, 126
isoflavones, 83
IUDs, 28, 30, 32
IUI. *See* intrauterine insemination (IUI)
IVF. *See*  in vitro fertilization (IVF)

joints, flexibility training and, 96

kidney disease, 29
Klonopin, 109
K-Y jelly, 158, 178–179

LDL. *See* low-density lipoprotein (LDL)
leiomyomas. *See* fibroids
LH. *See* luteinizing hormone (LH)
libido, loss of
    biological clock and, 167–170
    body image and, 164–167
    hormones and, 153–154
    lifestyle issues and, 159–161

medications and, 154–157
perimenopause and, 11, 15, 152–153,
    161–163
questions asked, 170–171
testosterone and, 158–159
unopposed estrogen and, 157
vaginal dryness and, 178–179
Librium, 109
licorice root, 80–81
life expectancy, 226–227
Loestrin, 47, 52, 58, 189, 197
low-density lipoprotein (LDL), 146–147,
    181–182, 190, 196
low-dose birth-control pills. *See* cycle
    regulators
lubricants, vaginal, 158, 178–179
lumps, breast, 133, 140
luteal phase deficiency, 168
luteinizing hormone (LH), 13–14, 168
lymph nodes, 133

mammograms, 59, 129, 130, 144–
    146
medical care
    bimanual examinations, 141–143
    checkups, annual, 67
    doctor, communication with, 67
    doctor, when to call, 33, 59
    future developments, 223–228
    getting the most from, 136–138
    Internet, as information source, 201–
        209
    knowledge as power, 211–222
    managed care, 136–138
    managed care and, 136–138
    pelvic examinations, 27, 141–143
    physical examinations, 139–140
    questionnaires, answering, 138–139
    questions asked, 151
    testing, need for, 141–150, 151
medications. *See also* hormone replacement
    therapy (HRT); tranquilizers
    libido changes and, 154–157
    night sweats and, 40
    side effects, 38, 41, 43–44, 56
    weight-loss preparations, 101, 103
Medline, 208
medroxyprogesterone acetate, 60, 195
melatonin, 108
memory loss. *See* forgetfulness

menopause. *See also* blood tests;
  perimenopause
  age of onset, reaching, 19–20, 21,
    172–174
  birth-control pills and, 64–65
  defined, 19–20, 172
  heart disease and, 180–182
  questions about, 186–187
  support/support groups for, 201–209
  surgically induced, 175, 180
  symptoms, 32, 174–178
  urogenital changes of, 178–180
menstrual calendars, 28, 138
menstrual cycle. *See also* abnormal bleeding;
  birth-control pills (BCPs)
  cramps, painful, 33–34, 115
  hormonal function and, 13–14, 25–26
  midcycle spotting, 28, 29, 45, 59
  perimenopause and, 11–12, 23–33, 45
  periods, absent, 26–28, 172–173
  periods, heavy, 30–31, 59
  periods, irregular, 11, 31–32
  periods, light, 32–33, 47–48
  periods, longer than usual, 28–29
  periods, missed/missing, 24–27, 45
  periods, twice a month, 29–30
metabolism, changes in, 89–90
methyltestosterone, 158, 159
Metrodin, 168
midcycle spotting. *See* menstrual cycle,
  midcycle spotting
migraine headaches, 39–40, 114–115
miscarriage, 28, 30, 169
mood swings
  causes, 15, 37-38, 65–66, 95, 196
  treatment, 103–106
motherwort, 81
Motrin (ibuprofen), 115
MSG, 40
myomas. *See* fibroids
myomectomy, 126

natural remedies
  depression, 113
  guidelines for, 81–83
  questions about, 84–86
  risks of, 68–72
  specific preparations, 72–81
nausea and vomiting, 34, 39–40, 114, 115
nervousness. *See* anxiety

neurotransmitters, 38, 112, 113–114, 225
night sweats, 40, 177–178
nipple discharge, 27, 34
North American Menopause Society
  (NAMS), 206
nutrition, good, 66–67, 76, 83, 117, 130.
  *See also* body weight

Ogen, 193, 194
omega-3 fatty acids, 76–77
oral contraceptives. *See* birth-control pills
  (BCPs)
Ortho-Cyclen, 50, 53, 55, 59–60, 189
osteoporosis
  causes, 97–98, 182–184
  prevention, 190
  risk factors for, 184–185
  treatment, 185–186, 197
ovarian cancer, 54, 63, 128–129
ovarian cysts, 54
ovaries
  function, 167–168
  menstrual cycle and, 13–14
  surgical removal of, 21, 175
overeating, compulsive, 117
over-the-counter medications. *See*
  medications
ovulation
  anovulation, perimenopause and, 12, 14,
    17, 25, 49
  identifying time of, 17
  pain with, 21–22

Pap test, 29, 141, 147–150, 151
parathyroid hormone, 183
partial hysterectomy, 134–135
patches, skin, 193–194, 198, 199
Paxil, 109, 112, 113, 114, 155
pelvic examinations, 27, 141–143
pelvic infections, 28–29, 30
pelvic inflammatory disease (PID), 33, 55,
  167
Pergonal, 168
perimenopause
  anxiety and. *See* anxiety
  breast soreness and. *See* breast soreness
  cramps and, 33–34
  depression and. *See* depression
  diagnosis of, 15–17
  forgetfulness and. *See* forgetfulness

perimenopause (*cont.*)
    headaches and. *See* headaches
    libido, loss of, 153–154, 171
    menopause, compared to, 18, 19–20,
        68–70, 83
    menstrual changes of, 23–33
    mood swings, 38–39
    natural remedies for, 68–86
    onset of, 19–21, 22, 172–173
    PMS, compared to, 44
    pregnancy during. *See* pregnancy
    sleep disturbances and. *See* sleep
        disturbances
    symptoms, 10–11, 14–18, 26, 45, 48–
        53
    symptoms, psychological, 35–43
    treatment, 48–60
periods. *See* menstrual cycle
phenylpropanolamine, 102
phlebitis, 56
phytoestrogens, 70, 72, 83. *See also* natural
    remedies
PID. *See* pelvic inflammatory disease
    (PID)
Pill, the. *See* birth-control pills (BCPs)
pituitary gland, 13–14, 26, 27, 30, 147
"plant estrogens," 70, 72, 83
PMS. *See* premenstrual syndrome (PMS)
polyps, 28–29, 120, 127–128
precancer. *See* hyperplasia (precancer)
preferred provider program (PPO), 136
pregnancy. *See also* birth-control pills
    (BCPs)
    ectopic, 54
    light periods and, 32
    miscarriage, 29, 30, 169
    during perimenopause, 20, 24–25,
        167–169
Premarin, 64, 179, 191, 193, 194
premature ovarian failure, 186–187
premenstrual syndrome (PMS), 44–45,
    61–62
Prempro, 195
progesterone. *See also* birth-control pills
    (BCPs)
    breast soreness and, 34
    depression and, 113–114
    lack of, physical symptoms, 14–17
    menstrual cycle and, 13–14, 25, 59–
        60

replacement therapy, 53, 189, 194, 196,
    199
    testing for, 26
progestins, 60, 128
prolactin, 26
prolapse, uterine, 124
Prometrium, 194
prostaglandins, 34, 79, 115
Provera, 60, 194
Prozac, 113, 155
psychological symptoms of perimenopause,
    15, 35–43
pulmonary emboli, 56, 198

raloxifene, 129, 196–197, 224
Replens, 158, 179
Restoril, 35
rheumatoid arthritis, 55

Saint-John's-wort, 113
saline-infusion sonohysterography. *See*
    sonohysterography
salt intake, 14, 62, 67, 94–95, 195
selective estrogen receptor modulators
    (SERMs), 64, 196–197, 224
Serophene, 168
serotonin, 38, 112
serotonin reuptake inhibitors, 113–114
Serzone, 113, 155
sex drive. *See* libido, loss of
sexual intercourse, 32, 55, 135
sexually transmitted diseases (STDs), 33,
    135, 167
skin, estrogen and, 189, 190
sleep disturbances
    causes, 15, 21, 37, 40–41
    treatment, 106–108
sleeping pills, side effects, 35
smoking
    birth-control pills and, 56, 64
    cervical cancer and, 135
    cessation, 66
    menopause, age of onset and, 21,
        172
sodium. *See* salt intake
sonohysterography, saline-infusion,
    121–122, 126, 128, 131–132, 134
soy, 78–79, 85–86
spotting. *See* menstrual cycle, midcycle
    spotting

STDs. *See* sexually transmitted diseases (STDs)

stress
anxiety and, 110–111
forgetfulness and, 116
hot flashes and, 175, 176
libido, loss of, 160–161
missed periods and, 25, 45
reduction, methods of, 66
sleep disturbances and, 107–108

stroke, 49, 200

support groups, menopause and, 206, 218

surgery. *See also* dilation and curettage (D&C); hysterectomy
fibroids and, 124–127
polyps, 127–128
questions about, 131–135

sweating. *See* night sweats

testosterone, libido and, 158–159

theophylline, 106

thyroid gland
anxiety and, 41
calcium metabolism, role in, 183
menstruation and, 26, 29, 30, 32, 172
perimenopause and, 15

total hysterectomy, 134–135

tranquilizers, 32, 35, 109–110, 112–114, 155

transdermal estrogen. *See* patches, skin

transition. *See also* perimenopause
diagnosis of, 18–19
mental attitudes toward, 211–222
symptoms, 12, 65, 87–98, 153–154

transvaginal ultrasound. *See* ultrasound, transvaginal

triglycerides, 146

tryptophan, 105

tumors. *See* cancer; fibroids

ultrasound, transvaginal. *See also* sonohysterography
benefits of, 141–143, 225
fibroids, 231
images, examples of, 230–232
ovarian cancer detection, 129
polyp detection, 230
postmenopausal bleeding, 29
uses of, 17, 19, 26, 230–232

unopposed estrogen. *See* estrogen

urinary symptoms, 126, 179–180

urinary tract infections, 180

urogenital changes of menopause, 126, 178–180

uterine cancer. *See* endometrial (uterine) cancer; hyperplasia (precancer)

uterine prolapse, 124

vaginal bleeding. *See* abnormal bleeding; menstrual cycle

vaginal dryness
causes, 18, 32, 65, 174
remedies, 157–158, 178–179

Valium, 35, 109

vitamin $B_6$ (pyridoxine), 62, 105

vitamin C, 180

vitamin D, 183, 186

vitamin E, 176

vitamin supplements, 67

Vivelle, 193

warts, genital (venereal), 135, 150

weight. *See* body weight

"withdrawal bleeding," 47

Xanax, 35, 109

yeast infections, vaginal, 155–156

Zoloft, 113, 114

zygote intrafallopian transfer (ZIFT), 169